PNT

Pain Neutralization Technique
An Unprecedented Revolution in Pain Management

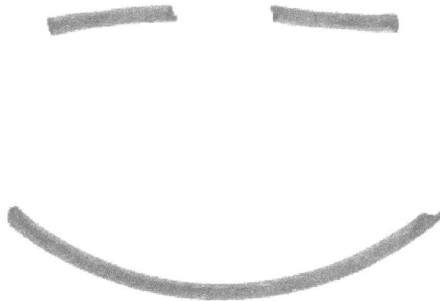

GASTON CORNU–LABAT, MD

WITH STEPHEN KAUFMAN, DC

Published by The 360 Home Group LLC.
15446 Bel-Red rd., Suite B-10
Redmond, WA 98052

This book may be available at special quantity discounts for bulk purchases for sales promotions, premiums, fund-raising, and educational needs. Special editions or book excerpts may be available to fit specific needs.
For details contact The 360 Home Group
360homegroup@gmail.com

ISBN: 978-0-692-47868-4

FOR ANA INES, FELIPE, ALFONSO AND PAULINE

With gratitude and certainty of the light

at the end of the tunnel

CONTENTS

DISCLAIMER, FOREWORD AND INTRODUCTION

PART 1

PART 2

Disclaimer: Calculating generally expected performance and results are difficult or impossible, because there is no "typical" patient or doctor. We've made a good faith effort to share the actual experiences of our practitioners and their patients. Every patient is individual in how they will respond to Pain Neutralization Technique™ treatment. Every practitioner (MD, DC, L.Ac, P.T., N.D. and L.M.T.) is unique in terms of their background, training, and understanding. Each will apply the procedures in their own unique way. Many patients with chronic and acute pain may show improvement. Some patients respond partially or do not respond at all. PNT and the other techniques are not effective for every patient. Several treatments are usually needed for lasting results. The reports in this book were all written by the doctors themselves; they may not reflect Dr. Cornu-Labat's or Dr. Kaufman's opinion. These are some of our best cases and may not be typical. Gaston Cornu-Labat, MD, Stephen Kaufman DC , and Kaufman Technique, LLC, and are not responsible for any loss or damage resulting from the use of anything written or implied in this book, or any of the Pain Neutralization Technique™ procedures. The Pain Neutralization Techniques™ are not for treatment of any specific disease or illness. No one should attempt any form of self-treatment using any of the information presented here. If you are ill, you should be under the care of a doctor. Very important note: in no case should any patient stop or modify any of their medication (or other medical treatment) without the direct consent of their own doctor!

More information can be found at:
www.painneutralization.com

Foreword:
Making the Impossible Happen

What you are about to read is truly astonishing, if understood correctly. Stories of hundreds of cases of people just like you and me (assuming you and I are anything alike). These people had chronic, long time pain and other symptoms, but were relieved unexpectedly, by simple, light touch, neurological reflexes. People in pain for decades for whom all other treatment had failed. Not just women, but men too. I would have trouble believing these stories if I hadn't seen many of them myself.

I teach my students to watch their patients' faces as they apply the Pain Neutralization Techniques. Most of the time, they see a startled look of surprise on the patients face, as extreme tenderness and pain that may have been present for years disappears on the spot when these techniques are applied. Patients are constantly shocked by this, and spontaneously blurt out *"Wow! That's amazing!"* without being coached. This phrase has become our anthem.

The doctors applying the techniques are every bit as surprised, even after years of practice.

The pioneers are the ones with the arrows in their backs.

Phrases like "Nothing can be done for you" and "You have to learn to live with it" lose their meaning here. The Pain Neutralization Techniques™ arose from my frustration at the ignorance of doctors who feel they know everything, to pronounce sentence on patients that they can't help (but maybe someone else can.)

For many years I had neck and back pain. The chiropractors and doctors I went to, even at chiropractic schools, told me there was nothing else that could be done for me.

They were wrong.

What they SHOULD have said was "I don't know anything that can help you- you've tried everything I know of. But keep looking- there are so many different techniques out there, something may help you."

As John Lennon so aptly said, "I used to get mad at my school, the teachers who taught me weren't cool." (If you were to study with me, it helps to be a Beatles fan.)

I was taught in school over 30 years ago that many patients with chronic pain could be helped, but I rarely saw it happen when I was in school, with what they were teaching. I saw some patients get temporary relief but need to go back for treatment again and again and again, with no lasting benefit.

If anything, most of these patients seemed to have a psychological addiction to treatment that provided very little real benefit. I thought that there must be a better way. There is.

With PNT we now have fortunately discovered so many ways to relieve pain, right away.

There's an old story about 2 doctors talking. One says of a 3rd doctor, "He's been practicing for 20 years." The other doc says, "NO, he's practiced the first year out of school 20 times, over and over."

Thousands of practitioners have eagerly learned the Pain Neutralization Techniques and applied them, with dramatic results you'll read about here. I am truly gratified by the response of both patients and practitioners to the procedures I've been fortunate to have stumbled upon. Every day I hear stories that make me happy.

In defense of the uninitiated, I must admit there is a lot of nonsense being taught in alternative health care. In ALL health care, for that matter. Yesterday's fads are today's banned, dangerous treatments. One **should** approach claims of a better method with skepticism and caution. I agree.

But I really make no claims. The procedures I've developed **don't** work for everyone. And mostly I let the doctors I've trained speak about their results. Please listen to what they have to say and investigate further.

Where there's this much smoke, there must indeed be fire.

When I said above "Making the impossible happen", I wasn't referring to treating incurable cases. That's easy. I was referring to getting health care practitioners to try something new, even in the face of overwhelming evidence that it's effective. Now THAT seems impossible! But it happens with everything new, not just in the health care field but in most places. At the end of the day I'm just glad to have been a part of this, and to have made so many friends doing what I love- helping people.

The other big obstacle we've had to overcome, is that I can't type. I mean at all. It's probably the single largest impediment to the spread of PNT My ideas and concepts are almost trapped in here! It's taken years longer than it should to get things done.

My 7th grade typing teacher actually failed me, the only poor grade I've ever gotten. Perhaps she's upset by my success, I don't know. I'm still trying.

Stephen Kaufman,DC

Denver, Colorado www.painneutralization.com

How this book came to be
Pain Neutralization Technique™ A holistic surgeon's discovery of an extraordinarily effective, non-drug, non-surgical, pain relieving technique.

During the fall of 2012, when my holistic and integrative medical practice at the Tahoma Clinic was getting started, I decided to expand my horizons and attend one of Dr. Kaufman's PNT Seminars.

Before embracing a holistic, general medical practice and joining the Tahoma Clinic in Seattle, WA, I practiced general surgery for many years both in academic centers and in rural settings. Regardless of the practice setting, the common factor for me has been the use of my hands in healing. With this in mind, it will be illustrative to read the feedback I sent to Dr. Kaufman one week after the seminar:

> *"The results are so astonishing I feel like a big kid in a BIG candy store. The results are so immediate and the technique so gentle that I find it addictive, I can't stop using it. For the last 20 years, until I joined the Tahoma Clinic and expanded my horizons, my specialty has been general surgery.*
>
> *My career has certainly been gratifying, but in essence, to relieve pain and suffering, I have to cause pain and suffering. This has been very present in my mind all these years. Now in many instances I don't have to. For me, as a healer, this is huge! What you have made available here Steve is mind boggling.*
>
> *As soon as I got back home from the seminar I went on a pain neutralization rampage with the clinic employees and practitioners. This rampage lasted 3 days and I treated about 30 people in between my scheduled work.*
>
> *One of our medical assistants had a couple of fractures and four subsequent surgeries in her right ankle about 10 years ago. She was told*

by her doctors that she would live with pain for the rest of her life and that it would keep getting worse. Pain pills would be the only option. She has lived with daily pain all this time. It's been 3 days now, the first 3 days in the last ten years that she has had no pain at all after I did some of the PNT techniques on her.

One of our receptionists has been dealing with carpal tunnel and epicondylitis symptoms (wrist and elbow pain) for 6 months. I treated her and when I asked her about it a couple of days later she said "Oh! I had forgotten about it!

Another patient had 3 years of knee pain after meniscus surgery and now is pain free after treating her with PNT in a 20 minute session.

I see huge potentials here beyond pain relief. What you have put together is remarkable. I think the most remarkable aspect of this is that it is crossing over "discipline" boundaries and I feel this may prove to be your most significant contribution.

*Irrespective of the uncertainty about the theories and explanations about how the techniques may work, **the reality is that PNT does work**. Consequently, this **should be a basic technique** for anybody that practices some form of healing art.*

During the seminar I felt a little overwhelmed by the amount of information and the significance I immediately perceived it has. On the other hand, the techniques were given in such an "organic" way that I was able to start hands on pain neutralization as soon as I got back to the Tahoma Clinic even without reviewing my notes and DVDs.

I received treatment from you and from other attendees during the workshops. My conditions were not particularly dramatic as in other cases that you demonstrated –I had low grade chronic lumbar pain and an annoying persistent pain/inflammation in my right knee after ligament repair and re-injury- however it was most remarkable to be able to experience the instant melting away of these tender points.

As we all know, experiencing on ourselves what we do to others most enriches our understanding. And, by the way, the nagging persistent "lights on" in my right knee is still gone (1 week later)."

As part of our initial assessment of the technique at the Tahoma Clinic I carried out a simple **uncontrolled study of the first forty patients that received treatment**, quantifying the immediate results after the first treatment. All patients scored their pain on a standard scale of one to ten, with "one" being very mild pain and "ten" being the worst pain imaginable. This **scoring** was done **before and immediately after treatment**. Twenty patients (50%) reported pain score of seven or higher before treatment. **Sixteen patients (40%) with "before treatment" pain scores of five or higher reported after treatment pain scores of zero or one. Eight patients (20%) had complete elimination of their pain with one treatment. Another eight (20%) had at least a five point reduction in their perceived pain score. All 40 patients reported a reduction of pain of at least two points**. Those who had partial relief with just one treatment returned for more. By the time the data compilation for the study was concluded **twenty three of the forty (57.5%) had complete relief of their pain**.

These results were the basis for the first article Jonathan V. Wright, MD, Tahoma Clinic founder and Medical Director, published in his well-known newsletter *Nutrition and Healing*. These results also were, albeit of the most basic kind, the first objective validation obtained regarding PNT They complement the experience I have collected treating patients, friends and family over the last two and a half years with extraordinary and highly rewarding results, and add one more layer of validation to the plethora of empirical evidence that is presented throughout this book.

My subsequent visits to Denver to learn more about PNT then added the remaining layers to cement a wonderful friendship with Stephen Kaufman. This friendship led to the idea of writing this book.

Given the state of affairs in the medical and healthcare fields (about which I share some pieces of my mind throughout the book), what best than to have an MD with almost 30 years in the medical field and a very broad range of experiences write "the book" about one of his most significant learning experiences in his medical career and about one of his most influential mentors in his medical practice who, by the way, happens not to be a medical doctor? Oh, my God! Is the world going upside down? I hope so and especially I hope with this book to be contributing significantly to that end within the healing arts; it's about time!

Cheers!

Gaston Cornu-Labat, MD
Holistic Physician and Surgeon,
Tahoma Clinic Redmond, Seattle, WA

Introduction

A lot has been published over the years about effective non-drug pain management. Many different techniques have seen the light, many are in use; many have come and gone.

None however can claim the miraculous simplicity and effectiveness of Dr. Stephen Kaufman's inspiration, Pain Neutralization Technique, or PNT.

Imagine for a moment that you have been suffering from knee pain for the last 2 years and it is getting progressively worse. Perhaps your actual situation is similar...

It started as an occasional twitch when getting up from your chair, after a couple of hours of working or reading. The weather sometimes makes it worse. You joke that you can predict storms. Then it became more frequent and went from an occasional, uncomfortable stiffness to a frequent dull ache that calls your attention at different times of your day and every now and then gets sharp. You start taking anti-inflammatory medication as needed. Over time you work your way up to a daily dose or two. Eventually even stronger pain pills become necessary to get you by and tune it down throughout your day. Your pain now is there every day.

At times the pain is worse than others. Maybe it's the weather, maybe that silly dance step you did the night before. Who knows? Yet pain is becoming part of your daily routine, pervasive; invading more and more of your mind with its presence. Recently, after some consultation with your primary care doctor, you have even been starting to entertain the idea of a knee replacement...

Using the knee as an example, such is the story of some 70 million Americans who are estimated to suffer from chronic joint pains[1]. In this example you happen to live in the Denver area, sometime around 2006.

One day while going for coffee at the office you grin when you reach for the sweetener and your typical nosy co-worker picks up on your discomfort and starts asking questions. You get annoyed, the pain issue has started to keep you on edge and sometimes -like today- it's worse than others. He is not a friend; you've barely seen him once or twice in the elevator. You are polite though, take a breath and mention your knee pain. "*Ohh...*" he utters, and then goes on "*Last week my cousin Vinnie told me about his hip pain and mentioned a Dr. Stephen Kaufman; he swears by him!*"

A very teenage "*...whatever...*" comes to your mind. You have been dealing with this for two years now, x-rays, prescriptions, the works... You smile and while you are working on putting the coffee pot back in place you mumble something like

"*Interesting...*"

---

[1] MMWR Oct 25, 2002/51(42); 948-950.

Yet the guy [proverbial nosy co-worker] still goes on "*He's a chiropractor out of Denver and has come up with something new for pain, apparently seems pretty amazing! Stephen Kaufman is his name, look him up...*"

You're bothered by having to discuss the subject of your pain yet you remain intrigued; something in his tone got your attention. Sometime later -on a particularly painful moment- you look Kaufman up and schedule an appointment. At this point you feel you have nothing to lose...

The day comes and there you are sitting in the treatment room. In comes this doctor, casually yet sharply dressed, polite but a little short. After a few customary questions and smiles, all the information that seems to have been pertinent is

"*...pain in my left knee... for about two years...*"

And then the PNT experience starts:

"*yeah, pain there... mmm... not now (ehh?)...*"

"*yeah, there too... better... mmm... gone (ehh?)*"

The motions repeat themselves, nothing uncomfortable, barely touching, some pressure, a few more times... five minutes later Dr. Kaufman is shaking your hand, telling you to see him again in a couple of days for another treatment. You get up and start finding your way out. You are still puzzled, not sure about what happened but, wait... your knee doesn't hurt...???...

Woww... that's amazing...

This expression literally bursts in your mind. Such is the story to which today thousands of people with one form or another of chronic physical pain can relate after visiting Dr. Kaufman or one of his many disciples that are now applying PNT on their patients with extraordinary success. Actually Dr. Kaufman has a group of posters ready on the side during his live seminars with expressions such as "WOW, THAT'S AMAZING!" Such expressions will burst out spontaneously, usually -at the most- by the third attendee/patient he treats during the very intense two-day PNT learning marathons. And, yes, the technique is actually taught to practitioners by relieving them of their own pain at the seminar; more about this later...

Since 2004 when Kaufman started teaching his technique, PNT has been slowly spreading far and wide throughout the US, and into Europe and Asia, and further south and east. Still, overall, a relatively small number of practitioners know about it or have even heard of it. Even less is the relative number of patients who could benefit from PNT and have actually heard about this God sent technique. Yet, it is coming and it's bound by its very nature to spread far and wide. This book's goal is to help along in this process. As you will be able to learn from the experiences presented in this book, given the tools available today for the management of pain, PNT is a true miracle and a blessing. Read on...

This book has been tailored in a very organic way to interest a broad audience. Some readers will engage this book with an interest and intention to find a resolution to their issues relating to pain, not being particularly interested on how, when or why. For these readers, jumping straight to Part 2 on page 41, where practitioners' testimonials start from the general to the specifics, will be the way to go.

These chapters can then be followed by Chapter 10 on page 75 where an indexed list of the broad categories or areas of the body where PNT has been found to be effective at present time are referenced, guiding to the subsequent chapters that present the specific reports. These reports speak for themselves. Getting a general idea about the PNT experience from chapters 5 through 10, then the readers can focus their attention to those areas of particular interest.

On the other hand, for those readers who are always interested in deepening their understanding and gaining the upper hand on what they are dealing with, for them starting with Part 1 will be the way to go. The book will walk the reader through an explanation of what PNT is and, to the best available knowledge, how PNT works, and a simple yet thorough explanation of what is known and understood about pain. This is then followed by a detailed recount of the history and context in which this wonderful technique saw the light. Finally the specific doctors' reports which attest to the effectiveness of this technique will follow in the subsequent chapters.

A good way to judge the quality of a non-fiction, educational book seems to be by the number of "Aha!" moments the reader will get from said book. It is the wish of the authors that this book will provide the readers with plenty of such moments.

PART 1

ABOUT

PAIN

NEUTRALIZATION

TECHNIQUE ™

Chapter 1
What is PNT?

Pain Neutralization Technique (PNT™) is **a new, unique, effective, and gentle way to instantly shut-off the pain signal to any given tender area in the body. In doing so PNT effects an immediate change in the tender tissue, and positively affects the cascade of events associated with those tender areas that lead to pain syndromes**.

PNT is the broad term coined by Dr. Stephen Kaufman DC, and used to describe a varied **series of gentle soft tissue maneuvers** that he discovered and developed. By using a number of very simple, gentle techniques by hand he is able to instantly **produce changes** in areas of palpatory pain. These changes range **from instant shut-off of the pain signal** (like throwing off a light switch) **to more subtle and cumulative changes leading** in many instances **to complete resolution or significant improvement** of the areas of pain, the associated pain syndromes and their other physical manifestations and symptoms.

PNT does not directly treat or press on trigger points or tender areas. While areas of palpatory pain are the target for this technique, **the work is not done on the tender areas themselves**. The work is **all done on the reflexes that resolve the pain in those areas**. This is the **cardinal difference between PNT and all other trigger point therapies** which press on or irritate the actual areas of tenderness (More on trigger points and areas of palpatory pain in Chapter 3).

The PNT procedures are **all neurological in nature; reflexes* innate to human physiology which, when properly elicited, shut off the pain signal to any given part of the body.** They work by **triggering** a neurological **reflex*** which causes an **immediate localized change** in muscle function and a consequent **elimination of the tender trigger point**; usually immediate or at times in delayed fashion. Because the treatment is neurological in nature, **very gentle pressure is necessary** so as to elicit the PNT reflexes and in most cases **just light touch** is all that is necessary for the desired reflex to be stimulated.

As previously mentioned, over the years a number of techniques have been brought forward to treat trigger points and their associated syndromes; *yet, until the advent of PNT no technique could claim to actually eliminate trigger points on the spot.* Often with PNT these areas of palpatory pain and the symptoms/pain they cause **do not return,** after just one or two treatments. In Dr. Kaufman's experience **with other methods,** trigger points would **remain tender after treatment** (like an uninvited guest at a wedding, Kaufman would say). **Relief** -if present- tended to be **temporary** and **frustrating** for the practi-

---

*Reflex – built-in involuntary nerve pathways that connect a given stimuli with a given action; for example the patellar tendon reflex: when the doctor taps right below the knee cap and the leg involuntarily kicks.

tioner due to the inconsistency of the results and the amount of pain the treatment itself often caused the patients. Last but not least, other techniques take their **toll on the practitioner**, wearing his or her thumbs out just from applying those techniques.

Also **PNT**, by its simplicity and ease of learning, **opens a large integrating therapeutic door** for many practitioners of very diverse disciplines; particularly for those coming from the so called *"conventional"* side of medicine (such as the author GCL) who tend to be very biochemically inclined in dealing with human body issues, and whose **understanding and integration of structure and function** has been limited, at best.

What Chiropractors and other "body workers" have known all along —that **structure and function are intimately related** in the human body- is now **accessible as a practical and easily applicable concept** to all practitioners of a broad range of disciplines. The integration of structure and function becomes **particularly evident** in areas such as the **viscero-somatic reflexes** discussed in Chapter 3 and, perhaps most notoriously, in pathological conditions such as hypertension (see also Chapter 3 and others).

Perhaps with even more significance, this **relationship between structure and function** also becomes **evident** in the reports of **issues relating to the gastrointestinal and respiratory systems,** where pronounced improvements in function are consistently seen with the treatment of related areas of palpatory pain (see Chapters 12 and 13). Some evidence relating to the central and peripheral nervous systems and the autonomic **nervous system** also contribute to reinforce this relationship between structure and function. Some reports of **"miraculous" resolution** of long standing, **"fixed" neurologic deficits** have reached Dr. Kaufman and are presented throughout the following chapters; also some of these experiences have been gathered by Dr. Kaufman himself.

Most important of all, no **adverse effects from this treatment have been reported so far**. While PNT is not effective in every case, **some degree of improvement** has been **uniformly reported** by all practitioners in the **great majority of cases,** and few are the patients that notice no favorable change at all. My own experience over several years confirms this. (GCL)

So, in summary, Dr. Kaufman drills repeatedly during seminars and other presentations what he calls "PNT Code of Honor;" the ten critical points that make his technique unique:

1– With other methods the treatment is painful and uncomfortable for the patient; the patient does not look forward to the treatment. The patient may bruise or quit after one treatment. **PNT is gentle, it is not forceful. Patients often say it feels good.**

2- With other methods the sore trigger point itself is treated. **PNT treats a reflex in the vicinity**, not the tender area itself.

3- With other methods the treatment usually doesn't get rid of the painful area, it is still painful at the end of the treatment. **PNT by definition is usually immediate.**

4- With other methods there is no immediate change in the trigger point. In PNT there needs to be instant reduction in the palpatory pain (not necessarily the symptom) in order to confirm the reflex. **Instant palpatory pain reduction is diagnostic of the adequate reflex being elicited.**

5- With other methods the treatment takes too long. **PNT takes from 5 to 90 seconds to find the correct neutralizing reflex, and 15-20 seconds to apply it.**

6- With other methods the treatment is hard work, hard on the practitioner; it is manual labor. Over time trigger point practitioners often develop repetitive strain injuries. They wear out their thumbs, wrists, shoulders, low back, etc. **PNT will save thumbs, wrists, and other joints; it is easy on the practitioner too.**

7- With other methods the treatment in mechanical. **With PNT, the treatment is neurological.**

8– With other methods too many repetitive treatments are required, and results are often not lasting. **With PNT four to six visits on average will often resolve most or all areas of palpatory pain.**

9– With other methods, the trigger point areas are still there, even after numerous treatments. Most other treatments don't actually make trigger points less sore or go away, although they may reduce the symptoms (spontaneous pain). **With PNT, after four to six visits, there are usually few or no tender areas left; and of course the symptoms are often resolved or greatly improved.**

10– Other methods treat only trigger points that radiate. PNT treats any tender area, not just the ones that radiate. Radiating points may have a higher therapeutic value but they are also easier to eliminate. **Radiating patterns usually end instantly with the correct PNT application.**

Chapter 2
Understanding Pain

Pain, in one form or another (except for some rare genetic disorders) is **experienced by everybody** alive. Hence, pretty much everybody alive knows from experience what the word *"pain"* feels like. Pain is the **most common reason for physician consultation** in the United States. It is also a **major symptom in many medical conditions**, and **can significantly interfere** with a person's quality of life and general functioning.

Agreeing that **everybody knows pain** in one form or another, a good question to pose would be **does everybody understand pain?** Pain can be understood as **a perception**. The International Association for the Study of Pain defines it as *"an unpleasant sensory and emotional experience associated with actual or potential tissue damage, or described in terms of such damage."*

For the most part in the general conception, pain is **understood as a signal in** some part of the **brain** that lights up in an **unpleasant** way when something somewhere in the **body gets hurt.** [See Figure 1 on page 17]

So, BANG! A thumb meets a hammer and a connecting cable (nerve) takes that BANG! to the brain where a red light goes on signaling PAIN from that proverbial hammer landing just off its intended target.

Well, this outline may be representative in an oversimplified way of what actually happens in the most simple of forms of the acute pain experience. However **the pain experience** is more complicated than this. Unlike the simple connection between the injury site (where the signal originates) and the brain (where pain is consciously perceived) with a cable carrying this signal (nerve); the pain experience is **actually multidimensional**. This means that in today's best understanding, many variables come into play when we experience pain.

Historically before the scientific revolution, pain was understood **as something originating outside the body**, perhaps —as the etymology* of the word points out- a punishment from a higher power. **As science progressed** in the understanding of the human body, starting with Rene Descartes in the 1600s, the understanding of pain went from a spiritual, mystical experience to a physical, mechanical sensation originated in the periphery of the body and ending in the brain. This understanding progressed through numerous purely **mechanical theories** until the late 20th century when things shifted again.

In 1965 Ronald Melzack and Patrick Wall introduced the **Gate Control Theory**. After a few years of fierce debate this theory became widely accepted. In short this theory now **placed the**

---

*Etymology of "pain" - First attested in English in 1297, the word *pain* comes from the Old French *peine*, in turn from Latin *poena*, "punishment, penalty" (also "torment, hardship, suffering") and that from Greek "ποινή" (*poine*), generally "price paid", "penalty", "punishment".

brain as an active system that filters, selects and modulates inputs from the periphery to generate the sensation of pain. Never again after this could anyone try to explain pain exclusively in terms of peripheral factors (i.e. injury to the tissues). [See Figure 2 on page 18]

By 1999 the **latest theory*** to explain pain surfaced, brought forward again by Ronald Melzack (Canadian psychologist and by then renowned worldwide authority in the science of pain). Known as "the **neuromatrix theory of pain**," it further refined the understanding of the role of the brain in pain.

In simple terms this theory explains the sensation of pain as the actions of a neuronal network (neuromatrix) "built-in" into the brain by genetic specification and "modified" by experience. **This neuromatrix generates the sensation of pain in the brain triggered by a variable combination of peripheral sensory inputs** (information coming from the periphery of the body through nerves), **inputs from different centers in the brain itself and the spinal cord**; and **affected by other factors as diverse as the immune and neuroendocrine systems, and the sociocultural environment** [Figure 3 on page 18].

In further understanding chronic pain, classifications have been proposed according to specific characteristics such as region of the body involved, system whose dysfunction may be causing

---

*R. Melzack. Pain Supplement 6 (1999) [s121-126]

the pain (e.g. nervous, gastrointestinal), duration and pattern, intensity and time since onset, and etiology. Other proposed classifications look at the type of pain such as nociceptive (coming from the nerve endings), inflammatory or pathological (due to inflammation or other problems in the brain itself).

Classifications aside, in dealing with naturally occurring phenomena such as pain, it always pays off to depart from established boxes and take a fresh look. After all, naturally occurring phenomena do not study books and other published technical literature before manifesting. Efforts to classify complex, multidimensional and incompletely understood phenomena such as pain will always fall short in their reductionism and in the authors' opinion should never be taken too tightly.

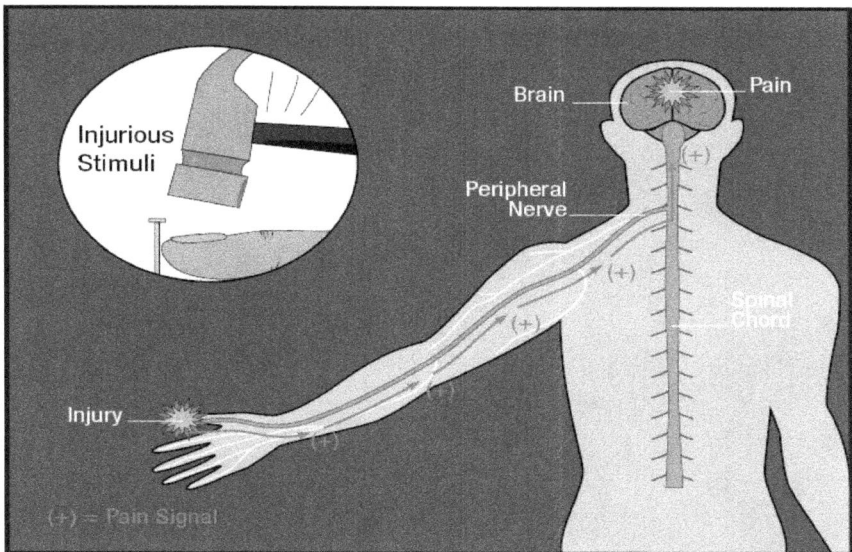

Figure 1- simple conception of the pain signal

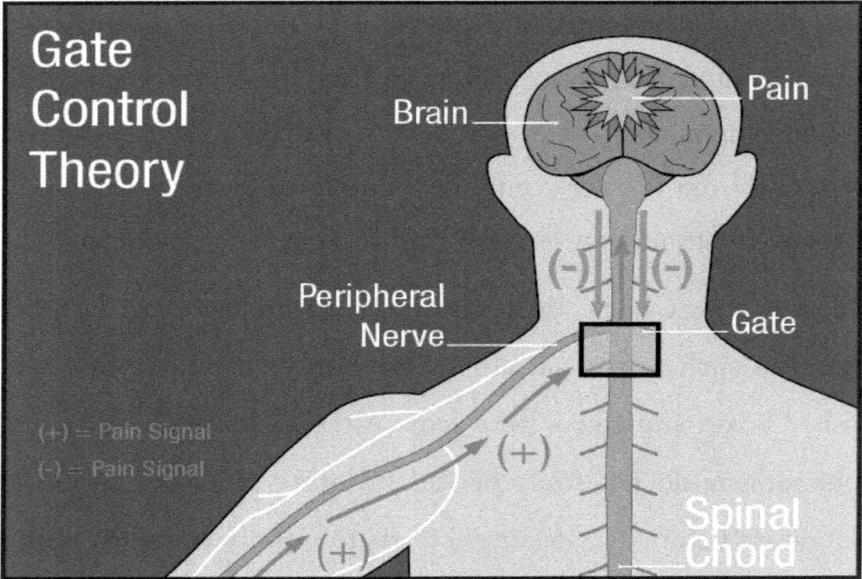

Figure 2 - Gate Control theory

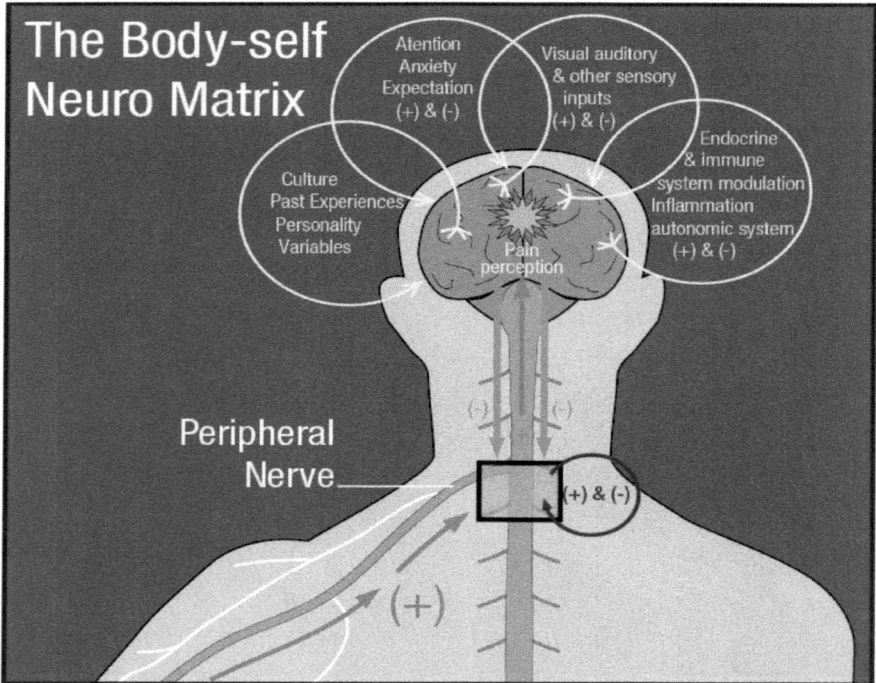

Figure 3 – Neuromatrix

Chapter 3

Myofascial Pain

Within the very broad world of pain, a **common source** of physical pain is known as **myofascial or musculoskeletal pain**. This would include most forms of muscle, joint, tendon, ligament, and bone pain. It was initially around these types of pain that PNT was first developed. Yet PNT has even broader applications.

Common types of pain syndromes that fit within the description of myofascial or musculoskeletal pain are **neck and low back pain, headaches, migraines, chronic joint pains such as shoulders, rotator cuff, knees and hips, iliotibial band syndrome and many others**. Syndromes such as sciatica, headaches, migraines, carpal tunnel, and temporomandibular joint disorder (TMJ) are frequently more closely associated with myofascial pains than with other pathologies such as scar tissue, chronic inflammation, x-ray changes, disk herniation, and other objective findings. Tennis or golfer's elbow, frozen shoulder and other such syndromes are often also associated with myofascial issues.

Published initially in 1983, Dr. Janet Travel, MD and David Simons, MD brought forward a major contribution to the understanding on myofascial pain with their 2 volume textbook: "Myofascial Pain and Dysfunction, the Trigger Point Manual."

Their most significant contribution probably has been the thorough description of the association between myofascial pain syndromes and what are known as **trigger points**. These are fairly consistent focalized tender areas in the myofascial tissues that somehow have a **causal relationship with pain syndromes**, and initiate and then perpetuate the associated syndrome.

Dr. Travell's (1901-1997) contributions to the field of myofascial pain management have been as significant as her career has been illustrious, becoming among other things the first woman to be appointed as physician to the President of the United States when elected President John F. Kennedy appointed her as his personal physician in 1960. According to Travell & Simons and others, trigger points are defined as an area particularly tender to palpatory pressure when compared to the same area in the opposite side of the body or to the surrounding tissue. A trigger point is possibly an area of localized ischemia or may be an area with some other localized changes in the tissue that promote a looped pain signal that remains on and affects surrounding and/or related tissues and structures. There are more precise and limiting characteristics of trigger points that Travell and Simons further established and that delineate what are known as classical trigger points:

- Pain on palpation of a discrete, irritable point in skeletal muscle or fascia, not due to local trauma, inflammation, neoplasm, infection or degeneration.

- A painful trigger point is palpated as a band or nodular area in the muscle; a local twitch response or "jump sign" may be elicited on manual stimulation of such point.

- Local palpation of the trigger point may reproduce the patient's symptomatic pain, and the pain radiates in a pattern specific to the muscle with the trigger point. Travell produced maps of the expected patterns of trigger point activity for every muscle in the body.

- Trigger point pain cannot be explained by neurologic exam findings or imaging studies.

Travell and Simon described several methods for treating trigger points, and since this major contribution, many techniques have emerged, been used and further developed over the years in efforts to treat these. Acupuncture, myofascial release, deep tissue massage, chiropractic adjustments are examples of the most commonly used techniques.

Results over the years have been variable with these techniques, both in the resolution of the symptom as in the duration of the improvement. Some other characteristics common to all these treatments have been observed and experienced by the Dr

Kaufman. As described in Chapter 1, with these previous methods (not with PNT) the treatment is generally painful and uncomfortable to the patient. Treatment is commonly applied to the tender area and is sometimes so painful that it discourages further treatment. Trigger points tend to remain painful at the end of the treatment with no immediate change to the area. These techniques also tend to require significant amounts of time and be hard work on the practitioner. Over time it is not uncommon for trigger point practitioners themselves to develop repetitive strain injuries, wearing out their thumbs, wrists, shoulders, or low back, since most of these techniques tend to be mechanical in nature. These techniques also may require a large number of follow up treatments to obtain lasting results and may only be able to address the associated pain without actually making the trigger points disappear. Therefore, patients may be prone to having their symptoms return.

As significant as classical trigger points have been, over the years it has been Dr Kaufman's experience that areas of localized palpatory tenderness that do not meet Travell's criteria are also significant contributors to a patient's pain syndrome. In particular, patients' problems may often be corrected when these "non-classical" trigger points are treated.

The understanding of this last concept —finding clinical significance to the so called "non-classical" trigger points- and its subsequent evolution led Kaufman to depart from this terminology. Today he teaches -and PNT practitioners generally re-fer to- **"areas of palpatory pain" (APPs)**. This conceptually rep-resents a **dramatic departure** from the limitations of classical trigger point definitions and, most importantly, **from all trigger point therapies**.

Although simple labels are being discussed here, Dr. Kaufman found necessary to emphasize this distinction because of the significant limiting preconceptions already associated with trig-ger points and classical trigger point therapies, and the obstacle these create. These preconceptions may influence in a limiting way potential patients that have previous less than satisfactory experience with trigger point treatment techniques. They may also influence (and in fact they frequently do) in a limiting way practitioners already versed in one or several of the many trig-ger point treatment techniques previously developed over the years, leading them to dismiss the opportunity of learning something truly revolutionary.

3 Types of Pain

In further understanding myofascial pain, another important clarifying note always emphasized by Dr. Kaufman is in under-standing the difference between **subjective** or spontaneous per-ceived pains (the patient's symptom, i.e. shoulder pain, neck pain, low back, wrist, etc.) and palpatory or **objective** pains (broadly labeled as APPs). In the PNT practitioners' experience there is a high correlation between elimination of an APP and improvement or resolution of the patient's symptom. In other words, addressing and resolving the objective components of the pain syndrome —even if not exactly located where the pain is perceived- will improve or resolve the subjective or spontaneous perceived pain: the patient's symptom.

A good example to illustrate this last point comes with the common occurrence in patients with complaints of wrist pain — not uncommonly labelled "carpal tunnel"- who are found to have tender areas in the elbow. With these then being subsequently treated (in the elbow), the patient experiences resolution of the wrist pain [SK, GCL and others experience].

A third broad functional type of pain that Kaufman likes to differentiate from palpatory or objective, and spontaneous or subjective, is **pain on movement**; pain that occurs on motion when muscles, tendons, and ligament in joints hurt when the patient moves the joint or group of joints in question. This type of pain also has a strong association with APPs and often resolves when these are adequately treated. Pain on movement may also resolve at times when the painful movement itself is treated with the appropriate reflex (more on reflexes also in Chapter 3). In Dr. Kaufman's experience establishing clearly a distinction with each patient between these 3 types of pain is an integral part of a successful treatment.

In summary, through large collected practical experience and - to this day- more than 6000 papers published in the medical literature on myofascial trigger points, there is well established symptomatic causal relationship between areas of palpatory pain and subjective, spontaneous or motion pain.

Using the previously established (pre-PNT) terminology, although little is still understood regarding the actual cause of trigger points, trigger points are now widely accepted as being a major cause of chronic myofascial pain. Going further from this last concept, with the advent of PNT and its evolution, classical trigger points and their significance is being broadened conceptually to give significance to any area of palpatory pain in the face of a much larger number of associated pain and functional syndromes. In other words, a lot more than what was previously known and accepted can now be accomplished by effectively treating areas of palpatory pain.

Areas of Palpatory Pain

Although less well established in the scientific literature than the symptomatic causal relationship just reviewed regarding trigger points and myofascial or musculoskeletal pains, similar associations are found through the collected experience of PNT practitioners between APPs and pain syndromes such as post-surgical pain. This is a not uncommon and certainly undesired complication of surgical procedures such as, for example, hernia repair or abdominal surgeries. Other surgical interventions such as orthopedic repair of fractures or amputations commonly present with related residual chronic pains (phantom limb pain is a good example) that are found to have associated areas of palpatory pain and, most importantly, can find resolution when these tender area are adequately treated, through PNT the results are often startling and immediate.

The observed association and the exploration of these potential correlations between any given physical manifestation of pain and areas of palpatory pain is in part what took Dr. Kaufman to depart from the trigger point terminology and its preconceptions, and adopt the APP terminology. This also led to the exploration of the effects of neutralizing any area of palpatory pain to evaluate its effects on any given manifestation of pain. Finally, this opened a huge door for PNT to -both conceptually and in practicality- grow and expand from a trigger point therapy into, potentially, a discipline in its own right. PNT is certainly becoming a complementary discipline with very broad applications in many health related specialties, and with an enormous potential [see Part 2].

Other Pain Syndromes and Functional Disorders Found to be Associated with Areas of Palpatory Pain

In a similar fashion mounting experience among PNT practitioners is finding associations between effective elimination of areas of palpatory pain and functional disorders of the gastrointestinal and genito-urinary tracts, respiratory system, central, peripheral and autonomic nervous systems, and other organ systems.

These observed associations range from resolution of chronic abdominal pain, nausea or irritable bowel syndrome, to marked improvements in functional lung capacity in chronic and acute pulmonary dysfunction and asthma, improvements in hypertension, eyesight and hearing, sleep, and fatigue and low energy states, among others.

These associations, at least in part, are understood to be related not to a musculoskeletal origin but to viscero-somatic reflexes (VSR) manifesting as areas of palpatory pain. These APPs are understood to be a manifestation of areas of dysfunction or problem with viscera. By affecting these somatic manifestations PNT has been found to affect the function of the viscera that is manifesting through this tender area. Through a reversing signaling or countersignal on these reflex pathways, bowel, respiratory, and uterine function, menstrual symptoms, asthma, some components of COPD (chronic obstructive pulmonary disease), and lots of other issues can be corrected or improved by addressing these viscero-somatic APPs.

The collected experience at this point is based on a large number of anecdotal reports to Dr. Kaufman coming from practitioners and patients. These case reports open the doors to very exciting possible therapeutic applications and to furthering the understanding and management of complex medical problems that currently have little if any effective treatment options. Complex, poorly understood, and difficult to treat pathologies such as tinnitus (chronic and persistent ringing in the ear), headaches and migraines, fibromyalgia, reflex sympathetic dystrophy, peripheral neuropathies, and others are among a number of these types of problems that have been reported in many instances to respond favorably to PNT treatment. More information can be found in this regard further along in the index in Chapter 11 and corresponding other chapters.

Chapter 4

The PNT Story

How did PNT Come About?

Every significant contribution in medicine, and likely in science in general, has always required the contributor to view any given problem in a new light, to think "outside the box" as it is commonly said. Einstein clarified this point exquisitely in one of the quotes he left behind, "*a problem cannot be resolved with the same kind of thinking that created it in the first place.*" Likely the same as every other contribution in the history of medicine, personal motivations also have always played a role in the stimulation of the "outside the box thinking" so as to tackle any given and unresolved problem. In the case of Dr. Stephen Kaufman and the story behind the advent of PNT, well... the story is no different.

Dr. Kaufman candidly recounts his "constant pain experiences" as a child growing up in New York City. Although he was very active, he was not —in his own description- a "natural" athlete and would often suffer injuries to shoulders, elbows, wrists or knees. As a teenager he avidly pursued martial arts. Bruce Lee was his hero and he was planning to become "*Lee's Jewish equivalent!*" He worked out 3 to 4 hours a day and succeeded both in obtaining several belts, and in developing a low back problem that stayed with him for 25 years. Today he reflects about this back pain having been a good thing for him since he came to realize early on that the medical profession had little to offer in this regard; and consequently this giving rise to the necessary "outside the box" thinking process.

Kaufman started practicing yoga daily by age 18. While he gained impressive flexibility, this discipline did little for him regarding his back pain. He also started visiting chiropractors at a young age. On his first experience in Buffalo, NY, the adjustments were forceful and counterproductive, and highly unpleasant to him. However, he did develop a habit of "cracking" his back to self-adjust it. Today he strongly discourages this self-treatment practice as most detrimental.

A few years later in Northern California, when dealing with a particularly challenging hatha yoga posture, he injured himself once more. This new injury led him to visit another chiropractor in the hopes of some desperately needed relief. This time his experience was much different with gentle adjustments together with some additional soft tissue techniques that accomplished in three consecutive visits a significant resolution of that injury. This experience was to change the path in his life. He became a chiropractor. Not only was he interested in learning about the adjustment of hard tissues (bones, cartilage and joints) but in learning about soft tissues which, in his opinion and experience, bore quite a bit of significance in most pain problems.

Throughout chiropractic school Kaufman was able to observe adjustments being used over and over to address pain syndromes with variable results. Although some patients obtained long lasting relief from chiropractic manipulation, in his observation these were a minority of cases. It was obvious to him that there was more to the equation than simply "cracking backs." He recalls other students sharing similar impressions and remembers how they use to congregate, *"...clump together and hang out, sharing stuff we had learned at seminars, oohing and aahing at the miracles of the human body we were discovering..."*

By the time Dr. Kaufman graduated from chiropractic school his back *"was a mess."* He had almost constant back pain. This was not only painful but humiliating! *"Here I was, a licensed chiropractic doctor, a supposed expert on back pain!"* He has observed this "paradox" in hundreds of chiropractors over the decades.

In his insatiable quest for his own pain relief and consequent best possible treatment for his patients, Kaufman furthered his studies on acupuncture and acupressure. Although interest in this discipline had been present for him from early on, while in chiropractic school, acupuncture was not a well-established discipline in the USA and was not practiced outside of the Asian communities, being there no accredited schools in the country yet. Eventually he studied with several teachers and obtained a certification in this discipline also. Yet this addition was not enough in his experience to address his own pain problems.

He also studied many other alternative approaches to chiropractic and soft tissue techniques including Applied Kinesiology, Sacro-occipital technique, Gonstead, Activator, Bennett, neurolymphatic, DNFT and cranial techniques, endonasal and myofascial release procedures, Nimmo's Receptor Tonus Method, strain counter strain, and a number of other trigger point techniques. Over the years he found these techniques valuable, yet his quest was not answered by any of them. After many years of practice he started wondering if there were some "magic switches" that could turn off these trigger points, just like a light switch.

In 1989 Stephen Kaufman formally set out on a research project to find this "Holy Grail," the ability to neurologically eliminate trigger points. His goal: ***discover some way to turn off trigger points and pain instantly***. His thought was that there may be a way to turn off trigger points without using mechanical pressure. Perhaps there was a way to stimulate neurological reflexes that would cause a muscle to change its functional characteristics or tonus in such a way that trigger points could be reduced immediately. It took more than a decade but he found first one, and then dozens of procedures that immediately deactivated trigger points.

The story goes that one day, while pondering on this challenging conundrum, he was lifting weights at the gym and lifted a dumbbell over his head to do a triceps exercise. The weight was heavier than he could handle. As he extended his arm, his triceps completely gave out; the weight and his arm plummeted towards the work out bench. Fortunately the weight missed his head; the PNT story could have been quite different otherwise. By using too heavy a weight he had triggered on his triceps muscle what is known as an inverse myotatic reflex (IMR), turning the muscle completely off. The weight had not slowly come down, it had dropped like, well... like a steel weight! He vividly recalls this being a very odd sensation. After this he reasoned that he had accidentally discovered a way to initiate an inhibitory reflex in his triceps muscle. He further hypothesized that if he could do that intentionally on a muscle that had a trigger point in it, then that trigger point might resolve immediately.

For Dr Kaufman a very important aspect of this insight was the fact that this was a reflex. In the case of this particular reflex, under certain circumstances when tension along a muscle becomes too great, the muscle relaxes, it "lets go." This is a defensive mechanism so that if too heavy a weight is picked up, to avoid tearing the tissue, this reflex is triggered and the muscle relaxes completely. This reflex is also known by other names, such as the Golgi tendon organ reflex. Like the patellar tendon reflex, this protective mechanism is part of the neurology of the muscular system.

The fact that this phenomenon is an inborn reflex, as mentioned before, is important. Since it is a reflex, it is natural for the body to respond in a predictable way. Although the response may vary in intensity from person to person, it is consistent in being present.

This significant insight then paired up with a parallel observation in regards to neck and upper trapezius muscle pain (the muscle joining the shoulder and the neck). It had been Dr. Kaufman's experience that when doing a certain procedure in patients' necks it consistently eliminated a certain type of pain in the neck and the trapezius area. He reasoned then that he had been triggering an IMR reflex with his neck procedure that eliminated a problematic trigger point in the trapezius muscle. From this point on, careful experimentation and observation with subsequent patients gave rise to the first of many of Dr. Kaufman's discoveries that originated the technique we know today as PNT.

2004 was the year when Dr. Kaufman started teaching PNT to other practitioners after laying down the basis for what he calls "the local reflexes." These local reflexes are the early, initial PNT developments; those reflexes elicited in the proximity of the APPs being treated. These were the first set of reflexes Dr. Kaufman discovered. Then came the manual spinal reflexes; broadening the impact and reach of each reflex by being elicited at a more central location near the spine. These were an intermediate step in the PNT development and this set of reflexes further broadened the spectrum of pathologies that respond to PNT The most recent developments have been labeled cranial or subcortical reflexes. Again, by having a more central location, they further broaden PNT's scope and effectiveness. In addition to rapidly eliminating pain, the spinal and cranial reflexes also greatly enhance overall functioning, often producing euphoria, a deep sense of well-being, greater energy, etc...

The 2007 A.C.A.M. Meeting
How the Word About PNT Started Getting Out
Into The Medical World

A key event in the history and evolution of PNT took place at the 2007 Annual Meeting of the **American College for Advancement in Medicine** (ACAM). This meeting was seminal in getting the word on PNT out into the medical community. ACAM is an international organization of medical practitioners going on 40 years of service. It is the strongest voice of the safe and effective practice of integrative medicine and nucleates about 800 integrative medical practitioners from 30 different countries; including within its members many of the most prominent integrative medicine practitioners in the USA.

The story goes that sometime in 2005 Steve Kaufman got contacted by Dr. Terry Chappell, MD, Board member of the **International College for Integrative Medicine** (ICIM, another prestigious association that gathers integrative medical practitioners). Dr. Chappell invited him to talk at the ICIM annual meeting about his pain technique. By then Dr. Kaufman had started teaching PNT and the word was slowly starting to get out.

Dr. Kaufman gladly accepted the invitation and prepared for the event. As the date approached he recalls getting nervous about the event, "*as a chiropractor talking to medical doctors I wasn't sure how I would be received...*" Kaufman had then already been doing PNT for several years. Yet he had not realized then that patients commonly had immediate and many times dramatic symptomatic improvement. His practice to this day includes not asking immediately after treatment about the results. Since at times relief takes a while to set in, immediate questioning right after treatment may create for the patient false expectations and unnecessary disappointments. Because of this Kaufman always stresses his recommendation not to ask patients about results upon completion of the treatment but to trust the technique and do the follow up in one or two days. Because of this routine, Kaufman was not fully aware at that time of the immediate and dramatic improvements that frequently are accomplished with PNT. This said, getting ready to talk about his pain technique at ICIM he thought he could get some immediate results right on the stage and make a significant impact on the audience. Still he was nervous and seriously considered running away *"tell them I got dysentery and couldn't make it..."* Yet he decided to stick to it.

As the presentation got going and after the appropriate introductory explanations, Kaufman started inviting participants from the audience for treatment right there on the stage. One of the first participants to come up was Dr. Ted Rozema, a well-known integrative medical doctor (who at the time Kaufman had not met). Dr. Rozema had been suffering from chronic back pain for about 30 years, which was instantly relieved by Dr. Kaufman's techniques (see Dr. Rozema's testimony on page 66). Kaufman identified and eliminated several areas of palpatory pain in his back and Dr. Rozema went back to his seat. While moving along treating other participants, Dr. Kaufman could see Dr. Rozema in the back of the room in very animated conversation with Dr. Robert Rowen, MD, Editor in Chief of "Second Opinion" Newsletter, the second largest integrative health periodical newsletter in the country.

By the end of the presentation several participants spontaneously volunteered that their longstanding chronic pains had completely resolved by the end of the presentation. It was at this point that Dr. Kaufman fully came to terms with the dramatic effectiveness of his technique. A report of what was witnessed at this ICIM meeting is what Robert Rowen would latter publish in his newsletter Second Opinion in 2006 as the first published article in a health magazine featuring Dr. Kaufman and PNT (see Dr. Rowen's testimony on page 66).

All this was the preamble to the ACAM Convention in Phoenix, AR in November of 2007. Dr. Kaufman submitted an application to present his technique at this meeting. Because of the influence of well-known integrative practitioners, including Dr. Rowen, Dr. Rozema and Dr. John Trowbridge, he got accepted almost immediately.

His presentation took place first thing in the morning on the second day of the convention. It happened in front of about 325 participants. Kaufman talked for about 45 minutes and then asked for volunteers. The first participant to volunteer had a painful point in his upper trapezius (very common) and responded in less than 30 seconds; *"pandemonium broke loose when I did that..."* Kaufman recalls. *"Rob Rowen stood up and positioned himself right beside me to watch, and a bunch of volunteers jumped up with all sorts of pains to be treated..."*

From that historical meeting he further recalls *"I have no idea what I said at the presentation but when I walked out a dozen doctors walked right behind me asking to be treated and a massage table materialized out of nowhere. Rob Rowen and his wife Dr Terri Su stood right by me the whole time and I continued treating people until 11 PM that night."*

This scene was the one Jonathan V. Wright, MD (Founder and Medical Director of the Tahoma Clinic) and his wife Holly walked right into and witnessed. This certainly sparked Dr. Wright's interest. It would be this interest which would later lead him to invite the author (GCL) to participate in one of Dr. Kaufman's seminars in 2012 and then lead to this point.

"Rob Rowen, Terry Chappell and I just had a great time with this and many people got relief or cure from their chronic pain issues. Then is also when I met Dr. Hyla Cass and we became longtime friends" Kaufman further recalls. He had the presence of mind at the time to ask from every participant who experienced his technique for a testimonial. This collection of testimonials and the subsequent publications that followed, again in Second Opinion, and later on in Nutrition and Healing (Dr. Wright's newsletter) ***"gave a huge rocket push to PNT in terms of acceptance in the medical community. Likely there had never been a situation where MDs had been exposed to a non-pharmacological soft tissue neurologic technique that produced instant and in many instances long lasting or permanent relief of pain."***

PART 2

PRACTITIONERS'

EXPERIENCE WITH

PNT™

Chapter 5
What Practitioners have to say about their experience with PNT

In terms of **significant contributions to the medical field**, at present time and with all of its tremendous potential for positive change, **PNT** is in its "infancy" barely coming out of Dr. Kaufman's genius, inspiration and dedication. As it comes out of Dr. Kaufman PNT starts **entering** into the **exponential growth phase** characteristic of all significant contributions to human knowledge. This exponential growth phase comes from multiplying the number of "heads" absorbing the knowledge collected thus far, interpreting and adapting it to each practitioner's experience, and then **expanding the collective** a little individual contribution at a time. It is this collective, when paired with an appropriate network that allows for effective sharing of all these individual contributions, the process which **brings forward significant paradigm shifts**.

There is no question in the authors' opinion, and likely in the mind of most readers, that **medicine** today, in one form or another, **is in dire need of major paradigm shifts**. A discussion about these needed shifts is beyond the scope of this book. Yet, processes such as PNT, are those that actually contribute to bringing these paradigm shifts. Enough to say here and now in regards to **PNT** that **effective non-pharmacological manage-**

ment of pain in its many forms, and the furthering of the integration of structure and function into the collective medical mind are two major contributions that Dr. Kaufman is bringing forward through this technique.

To this end and being this process at such an early stage in its development, what better than to share the collected experiences of practitioners worldwide. From the very inceptions of his PNT teachings Dr. Kaufman -systematically and very, very insistently- has been requesting all new and established practitioners for feedback and reports of their experiences with PNT At the time of this book's printing Dr. Kaufman had collected well over a thousand patient reports from more than 380 practitioner reports from diverse disciplines including medical, osteopathic, naturopathic, chiropractic, dental and veterinary doctors, acupuncturists, physical and massage therapists, registered nurses, etc...

Voluntary reporting of any given phenomena represents characteristically a small percentage of the actual collective experience regarding said phenomena. Even more valuable in the case of PNT is the fact that the majority of the reports presented throughout this book are not nameless objective clinical descriptions but the personal experiences of well identified practitioners all across the country and also from other parts of the world, who can be easily found and contacted.

With all this said, and starting with the own personal experience of "paining" practitioners, nothing is better than allowing "experience" to speak for itself. The reported experiences that follow are organized for either an entertaining and enlightening read, or to provide information focused on a specific area of interest based on the reported pain syndromes of particular interest to the reader.

The following chapters contain testimonials from prominent health practitioners which give general comments and descriptions about the technique. Next follow specific reports with an index at the beginning of chapter 10, loosely organized by body regions, reported pain syndromes, and other conditions that have been anecdotally or systematically found to response to some degree to PNT The reader can use this index to review the reported experiences for any area of interest. Most readers concerned with pain in one form or another will likely find at least one testimonial throughout the next chapters with which they will be able to resonate.

Important as a further disclaimer here is to point out that all reports published in this book are the personal recounts, experiences, and opinions of each individual named practitioner. These are their reports and while they may be typical, new practitioners' experiences may differ. Dr. Kaufman's opinions may differ also from those of the individual reporting practitioners. Also, the readers may notice at times an almost telegraphic literary style from some reporting practitioners, a style which is quite common among physicians and other healthcare workers in the process of documenting, describing and reporting their work. Being truthful to the reporting process, the author chose to respect for the most part each practitioner's style of communication as handed to Dr. Kaufman.

Chapter 6

Urgent Care MD finds in PNT a powerful tool for many patients

Jawad Bhatti, M.D is a physician in Midlothian, VA who is board certified in Pain Management and Physical Medicine and Rehabilitation. Up to the time of this publication Dr. Bhatti was practicing Internal Medicine as a Hospitalist, and in an urgent care center in Ferriday, Louisiana.

The following extraordinary case studies were submitted to Dr. Kaufman over a period of weeks by Dr. Bhatti. He had outstanding success with many conditions, applying the Pain Neutralization Techniques to many seriously ill patients. Evidently delighted and excited with his results with PNT, he provided Dr. Kaufman with a cornucopia of reports transcribed here as Dr. Kaufman received them.

Note: it was of course not possible to verify any of these extraordinary case histories, and the authors make no claim that people with similar conditions would respond as well. These cases have been included to show the wide range of people and conditions that may be helped with the various Pain Neutralization Techniques. Also many of Dr. Bhatti's patients had a disease or some form of pathology; in many cases PNT may not affect the pathology or the disease at all, but may still provide a measure of pain or symptom relief.

Also note that in many of these patients follow up reports were not available, so the authors don't know how long a particular result lasted. In many cases follow up reports are included, however. In no case should any patient stop or modify any of their medication (or other medical treatment) without the direct consent of their own doctor!

From Dr Bhatti:

> *"I work in an urgent care (federally qualified) public health clinic and I'm able to help a lot of people with the Pain Neutralization™ Techniques. They all are very, very thankful. "Wow" is the word I often hear.*
>
> *Using just the latest advanced PNT procedure; so far I've treated 49 patients for back pain with only 6 patients reporting less than 50% relief. (One of them had lung cancer which was metastatic to the hip.)*
>
> *37 patients were treated with neck pain and/or shoulder pain; only 3 of them had less than 50% relief. Most others had more than 90% relief. There were 2 fibromyalgia patients who had 100% relief. 5 patients had good relief of abdominal pain.*
>
> *7 headache patients had 100% relief.*
>
> *2 out of 3 patients with nausea had good relief.*
>
> *My observation is that patients who have knee and elbow pain along with neck and back pain also seem to improve. It starts easing off in about 5 seconds and takes about 10-15 seconds to reach the peak effect. A lot of my patients have restless leg syndrome and it seems to help that too.*
>
> *The low back pain PNT techniques worked on 3 patients with chronic back pain on narcotics to bring their pain down to a lev-*

el of 2 or 1- pretty impressive. One follow up showed her improvement maintained 4 weeks later."

Amazing Results in Hypertension!

"I've been getting amazing results for HTN. I've had numerous patients have very significant drops of blood pressure with one of the advanced PNT techniques. 13 out of 16 patients with hypertension had a substantial drop in blood pressure; the average BP in 11 patients dropped from 158/89 to 131/75! We'll follow up with these to see how long it lasts.

One patient with hypertensive urgency had a drop of 70 points systolic in 2 minutes! A follow up on this patient was that she did not have to go to the ER as her blood pressure numbers stayed low. Usually with symptomatic HTN urgency cases I admit them to hospital for 24 hours but in her case it was not needed.

I had another patient with BP 172/90 who dropped to 120/80 - please remember he has been on BP medication for 4 years and never been that low.

One lady with anxiety levels of 10 dropped to 0 in 20 seconds. She told me 'doc, it felt like I just took a tranquilizer!"

Pain relief in even severe osteoarthritis!

"I had a patient with knee pain from severe osteoarthritis with leg bowing. Using the Manual Spinal Nerve Blocks™ I was able to bring his pain down to zero. This amazed me. My nurse had plantar fasciitis. She got 85% relief from PNT and I was able to bring her heel pain down to zero with the Manual Spinal Nerve Blocks™. I used the advanced meridian bending for shoulder ROM on a patient with moderate to severe osteoarthritis, who had a complete range of motion increase from 90 to 180°.

One patient with severe osteoarthritis of the shoulder (who already had one shoulder replacement done) had 90% pain relief. I've had lots of other success stories similar to these cases.

Follow up on one of the patients with severe lateral knee pain and who was on crutches had an overall 80% relief with one treatment of PNT She's now walking without crutches and has cancelled her surgery."

Why do people use recreational drugs....?

"I just had a patient who left crying with happiness. She gave <u>me</u> an euphoric rush. She had severe knee pain for ten years. This was her second treatment and her pain was zero today for the first time in ten years. She has x ray proven moderate to severe osteoarthritis of the knees. I felt my endorphins releasing from this and I guess we all hope for these moments. I asked myself, 'why do people use recreational drugs .....they don't need them! You get much higher from seeing people so happy!'

I treated a patient for a clicking TMJ. The patient was shocked at the improvement, and left the clinic saying "its a miracle". I also used your meridian bending technique for panic attack and anxiety on a patient who had lost a child, with dramatic improvement. One patient had foot pain secondary to ankle fracture following an open reduction, internal fixation surgery a week ago. Her pain came down to 2 from 10 with manual spinal nerve blocks. The narcotic she was taking could only bring it down to 7.

I had a patient with rib pain secondary to severe coughing for 3 weeks who had an excellent response to the rib pull technique today. Another patient had severe myofascial pain for 5 years who comes in monthly. He had received trigger point and botox injections from me in the past. I applied PNT on him with 90 % relief in his neck and back on his first treatment today. He is on high dose narcotic medication but he did confess he's not felt like this in the last 5 years. I am planning to decrease his pain meds if his pain levels continue to stay down.

Patients with visceral dysfunction and pain

"I admitted 2 patients to the hospital last night, one with diabetes and sub-occipital abscess and the other with prostate cancer and prostatitis. I tried meridian bending on both of them for pain and it worked; narcotic pain meds only brought their pain down from a 9 to 7, but the PNT techniques brought it down to 1-2 (on a pain scale of 1-10).

A patient with chronic interstitial cystitis had 3 treatments from me so far and for the first time in 10 years her pain dropped to 0 after the 3rd treatment of a Manual Spinal Nerve Block™ and Visceral Impact Procedure™. She's very excited as her average pain scores have dropped so far and her functional life has improved a lot. Please note that she has tried acupuncture before with zero help.

I just had a patient with L4-5 paraspinal abscess with severe pain of 10/10. I drained the abscess and applied a manual spinal nerve block™ with 80 % relief. She had about 50 cc of pus which we were able to drain.

I had a patient with pain of 10/10 from a knee abscess. I gave him a manual spinal nerve block™ and his knee pain dropped to zero. Then I performed an incision and drainage on him. He's 27 years old and had back pain and carpal tunnel syndrome which also completely resolved with PNT So these techniques do work when there is pathology secondary to infection.

A cardiac transplant patient with fever of 101.6 dropped to 99.4 with meridian bending.

I had a patient with chronic testicular pain for 27 years on a high dose of narcotics,; after PNT Meridian Bending his pain decreased to almost zero from an average of 8-9. He was very happy and surprised before he left.

A patient with mastitis got 100% relief within a minute from a manual spinal nerve block. A patient with nephrolithiasis (kidney stones) also got 100% percent relief with a manual spinal block.

I just had a patient with 8/10 pelvic pain which dropped to zero with treatment.

PNT Visceral Meridian Bending so far had excellent outcomes on 3 patients with nausea and 2 more people with abdominal pain. Another patient who fell in a department store with severe back pain had very good outcome with one meridian bending treatment.

Another patient with breast cancer, following a mastectomy had severe pain at the site of the scar. Today her pain and ROM were zero, back to normal since the first treatment.

A follow up of 3 cases of carpel tunnel syndrome showed 2 of them treated with PNT reported 100% overall pain relief with one treatment at one month. The other patient is a physician with documented mild right and mild to moderate left CTS. The right side got 90 % relief with only mild relief on the left, 3 weeks after treatment."

Excellent results in respiratory and sinus patients and sleep apnea. Fevers drop in minutes. Vertigo disappears.

"Some cases which caught my attention today: an asthma patient who I've been treating for 1 year presented with wheezing and allergic rhinitis. She is on inhalant therapy. I utilized the respiratory techniques; with each procedure she felt she was able to breathe better and after the treatment I auscultated her and her wheezing was resolved.

Another case is a 9 month old boy who was on steroid therapy 2 weeks ago for possible brochiolitis. His mother also had a history of asthma and presented with wheezing, post nasal drip and rattling. I applied the same protocol as above on him and his rattling and wheezing significantly improved and his runny nose stopped. I placed him on the appropriate medications.

A physical therapist was having acute sinus pain and asthma exacerbation, and I tried meridian bending on her-in seconds she had immediate symptom relief and was pain free. The medication she was taking was not even close. I asked her to call me and let me know how long this lasts, and to keep track of how many times she has to use her inhaler. My 9 month old son was diagnosed with otitis media and on antibiotics and decon-

gestants. I tried meridian bending on him- after his first treatment his rattling disappeared and he perked up.

The temperature of a child dropped from 101.8 to 99.6 in a minute. A young boy presented with sore throat after a few days on antibiotic therapy. I tried the rublite on his throat with 100% relief of throat pain – his cough was also a lot better.

I saw a 2 year old child with documented fever of 102°, where the fever medication didn't work. I applied PNT and after 30 seconds her core body temp was decreased to 98°, measured by thermometer. I had a young girl with abdominal pain and fever secondary to urinary tract infection with nausea and vomiting, admitted last night. Her fever was 101.6 and she was very hot to the touch. After PNT her temperature dropped, she felt better and her body started cooling down instantly. Had another child with a temperature of 101.8° dropped to 99.6° after one minute of treatment.

A patient has been seeing me for 4 years with severe allergic rhinitis who takes at least 3-4 rounds of steroids per year. Today I treated her with a rublite on her sinuses with complete relief. She sounded very surprised.

I treated a dizziness patient with vertigo with your vertigo protocol- I saw him on a follow up today and he had tremendous improvement.

I treated a patient for sleep apnea and he had significant improvement in his symptoms instantly, with better breathing and he was not snoring as loudly. Please note that he had rhinoplasty done 4-5 years ago. Now the doctors were talking about another surgery as he not able to tolerate CPAP/BIPAP. His wife reported a significant reduction of sleep apnea after the procedures.

I had a gentleman with acute sinusitis and pink eye requesting a medication. I applied your rub lite procedure and the pain level of 10 out of 10 in the sinuses and eye dropped to 0 out of 10. His pink eye also had instant improvement. Another woman's sinus problem disappeared completely after using the rub lite procedure. I used your anxiety protocol with an excellent response on 2 patients."

Headache and limited range of neck motion of 20 years, gone!

I saw a patient who had severe headache and neck pain for 20 years with neck range of motion limited to only 20° on the left. He has been to every possible physician and chiropractor known to him in the last 5 years. PNT meridian Bending caused his neck pain and headache to go away instantly with complete active ROM, without any assisting. The guy left in surprise and happy, which made me happy. Please note he was here for his narcotic refills and was crying in pain before this procedure. Amazing....

I think meridian bending is a very powerful technique. 3 patients with headaches had complete relief from meridian bending between the scapula so far. One patient with nausea had relief with meridian bending."

Neuropathic pain, peripheral neuropathy, and phantom limb pain

"One lady with bilateral ulnar neuropathy had numbness as her major complaint. I did one of the upper extremity procedures on her and her numbness completely resolved.

I saw a 12 year old boy who was diagnosed with lumbar plexopathy 2 -3 years ago. This boy had only one session of PNT when I neutralized his psoas trigger point with the agonist technique. At that time I was in the initial phases of learning PNT My nurse called his home today and his dad is reporting 90% relief at one month, after just the one PNT application. His hip hiking is completely resolved. Please note he had an EMG at University of Jackson confirming the lumbar plexopathy diagnosis.

The lumbar plexopathy case is now off his muscle relaxant medication. He still has some back pain and tight hamstrings. I did the PNT Meridian Bending; he had significant improvement in his gait and started walking pain free. His flexion was 20° bilaterally at the hip with knee in extension before the treatment and became 90° degrees after the procedure.

I had a chronic inflammatory demylenating polyneuropathy (CIDP) patient scheduled today which has progressed to an ex-

tent where she was unable to walk. She is very reluctant to take medicines. She has received 2 rounds of IV gammaglobulins which gave her motor nerves some improvement. I did PNT meridian bending on her and she told me that it felt weird as it seemed her sensations were coming back and her burning pain had disappeared. She walked in with a cane and left without it. Please note the above diagnosis are confirmed and documented with serial NCS and EMG studies.

One 35 y/o patient with T1 spinal cord injury who's paraplegic has a bullet lodged in his neck with cervical radiculopathy and forearm pain bilaterally. He had 80% relief from manual spinal nerve blocks.

On a follow up the first patient I treated with PNT meridian bending for phantom limb pain reports zero phantom pain since the first treatment.

The thoracic outlet case was one of the hardest to treat but she had 50% improvement with 2 treatments. Her neck had minimal ROM but improved to 70° with the cervical protocol. A patient with bilateral severe epicondylitis got 90% relief. A patient with a hip prosthesis and knee pain had about 50% improvement with 3 treatments using combinations of joint repositioning and PNT.

A cervical and thoracic radiculopathy responded with 95% relief and in another patient I also had an excellent response. So far the rublite procedure has a 100% successful outcome with positive relief for sinus pain and ear pain- I've performed it on about 17 patients with favorable results.

I had a patient with diabetes and phantom limb pain of 10 (on a scale of 1-10) secondary to below the knee amputation. The pain level dropped to zero after the PNT application.

One patient who came at the end of the day yesterday had a history of diabetes mellitus, a recent coronary artery bypass graft, and burning pain in both feet secondary to peripheral neuropathy. I had him on neurontin but it was only helping when he takes it at night. I gave him a spinal nerve block with 100% relief of the burning pain. An 80 year old patient with breast cancer on chemo presented with bilateral breast pain; with a manual spinal nerve block it dropped to zero in 10 seconds; 20 minutes after the block she was reporting 2/10. A 34 year old MVA case with a concussion to abdomen, a severe hematoma on the left thigh and pain in the back of 10/10 dropped to 2/10 with a manual spinal nerve block.

At one month after treatment a spinal cord injury patient with neuropathy has still 100% relief; this is a very good outcome for neuropathy!

A patient with knee pain and tight hamstrings got 100% pain improvement. A patient with moderate carpal tunnel syndrome responded with 80% relief (after 1 treatment.) A calcaneal bursitis responded to PNT with 90 % relief.

Another patient with moderate CTS responded to joint repositioning of carpal bones with 80% relief. I tried the rub-lite for a patient and her sinus problems completely disappeared instantly.

I have a 25 y/o patient with fibromyalgia. I tried PNT and spinal blocks with an excellent response of 90% pain relief. She also has history of congestive heart failure and hypertension.

A patient with a displaced ankle fracture whose first cast failed and had recasting done last week with pain 9 out of a possible 10 dropped down to zero with a manual spinal nerve block. It seems like spinal blocks have very good response for acute pain with pathology. Please note I average about 40-50 patients a day in a typical month.

I did a follow up on a patient with low back pain who was disabled for 2 years with an average pain score of 9-10 with pain meds. On exam her case was more consistent with facet pain and possible radiculopathy. With one treatment of PNT and the low back techniques her score dropped to 2, on average. At her one month follow up today I did a cervical manual spinal nerve block™ and her pain dropped to zero. She's going to go back to work and got a work release from me. I also made her neck 20 years younger with the PNT cervical dynamic lift, which helped her headache to go away completely.

I had a patient with low back and leg pain with her whole side hurting, secondary to a CVA. Her pain levels dropped to 2 with a manual spinal nerve block™. A patient with moderate carpal tunnel syndrome responded to the extremity techniques with 80% relief. A retro calcaneal bursitis responded to PNT with agonist muscle technique with 90% relief. A patient with a displaced ulnar fracture got 70% pain relief with a manual spinal nerve block. The patient was referred for a surgical ORIF [open reduction and internal fixation].

A patient had fallen from a horse today and came to me with severe pain with bruised chest wall. A chest x ray showed a broken second rib. With the rib pull she had 75 % relief. I did not wanted to go further as I was concerned that further attempts may make her pain worse so put her on pain meds and told her to f/u.

I saw a 29 year old patient with a left below the knee amputation on narcotic therapy with severe hip pain and sciatica for years on the residual limb, and phantom limb pain on the left. He had a prosthesis which was few inches short. He got 100% percent relief on the sciatica 60% relief for phantom pain. I had a patient with sickle cell disease and chest pain and did spinal blocks with 80 % relief.

Another unusual case with forearm extensors shortening and tight tendons came today. This patient could not make a fist and had severe limitation of gripping bilaterally. PNT gave her 80% improvement, on the left, with 40 % improvement on the right.

A patient with fibromyalgia with severe back pain and bilateral leg pain responded with 80-90° relief with the manual spinal nerve blocks; then did the cervical protocol and she told me that she wants to take me home with her. I said no, I have other patients to take care of.

A patient with knee pain and tight hamstrings responded to traction and meniscal repositioning 100% pain improved. A patient with moderate carpal tunnel syndrome responded to the joint glides with 80 % relief.

Using the PNT procedures have certainly stimulated a lot more referrals, maybe more than I can handle. I have people who are now just coming for these procedures.

One patient who fell from a horse 10 years ago was on high dose of narcotic and tranquilizer therapy with severe limitation of hip flexion to 20°. PNT dropped her pain down to zero; with tears in her eyes she told me she's never felt pain free before, even with narcotics. Her pain score never dropped below 7. Her positive limited SLR before the treatment went to 90° of flexion. She will f/u in 2 weeks. A fibromyalgia patient with neck and back pain had 100% relief. Before the procedure she thought her pain was coming from her bones. She left very, very happy.

Another chronic back pain patient on follow up retained 60° overall relief after one treatment; for the first time, he knows how it feels to have no pain, as his pain dropped to zero after the 2nd treatment. He also left very happy. With time I'm able to benefit more and more patients, as I'm getting faster with practice.

The patient from 2 weeks ago with PNT meridian bending for low back pain is still reporting 90% relief at 2 weeks with one treatment. "

Ruptured quadriceps tendon, torn rotator cuffs, and a torn A-C joint

"I just had a patient with ruptured quadriceps tendon barely able to walk with severe pain above the knee. He had a visible deformity above the knee of the quadriceps tendon and ROM was limited on flexion, secondary to severe pain. Advanced meridian bending with knee flexion gave him 90° relief and he left my clinic on his feet walking pain free.

A patient with a Grade 4 AC joint tear with visual deformity of the shoulder responded to PNT with 78% relief. A patient with a severe rotator cuff tear with only 5 ° of movement was improved to 90° abduction on the first session with PNT At a 1 week follow up she still had 70° of abduction, up from 5°but decreased from 90° after her first treatment. PNT gave her another 40° degree of pain free abduction today. When I asked her if she wants any pain meds she said no. Please note she has not been able to do anything with this arm for the last six months.

Another patient, age 39, with a history of an auto accident who's been seeing me for 5 months with history of a rotator cuff tear and severe back pain. She'd received trigger point and botox injections in the past with minimal relief and is on narcotic therapy. I applied PNT for her back and a manual spinal nerve block™ for her shoulder with 90% relief. It seems like she was very happy.

Jawad Bhatti, MD Midlothian, VA
Board certified Pain Management, and Physical Medicine and Rehabilitation.

Chapter 7

Pain Management Specialist gets phenomenal results

John R. Baird, MD got introduced to PNT early on in its development. Since he started practicing this technique he has consistently provided Dr. Kaufman with a plethora of remarkable reports. Dr. Baird is a Diplomate of the American Academy of Physical Medicine and Rehabilitation and a former associate professor at the University of Tennessee in Chattanooga, TN. He practices as a physiatrist (specialist in pain management and rehabilitation medicine) in Louisville, KY.

From Dr. Baird:

> I've treated over 200 people using the PNT Techniques™. The most frequent response from patients is "that's amazing". I've only failed a few times to alleviate or improve folks (based on my experience I think those people had secondary gain issues for work related injuries or pain medications seeking). I'm so excited, since I having been practicing manual medicine now for over 15 years and have been searching for an easy, fast acting and effective technique. PNT is the answer, and needs to be used by anyone treating pain.

> As pain management physicians, we are under a lot of scrutiny now for our prescribing habits and your phenomenal techniques are the answer for me to transition to a hands-on treatment that is not hard on me, nor exhausting to do, with immediate amazing results. When you gave all the credit to God at the end of the conference that was the most moving part of the conference. The

advanced practitioners at the conference had some of the best hands I have ever had work on me.

I have had osteopathic, chiropractic, acupuncture, energy medicine, craniosacral and myofascial work and education by the best practitioners on the planet, and you have the most effective, immediate, and long lasting techniques I have ever experienced, seen or used on patients. I've practiced all of the techniques previously mentioned before I learned PNT and now I am a believer and will tell anyone willing to listen.

I've been able to relieve headaches, neck and low back pain, frozen shoulders, joint pain, jaw pain, carpal tunnel and radiculopathy instantly. Thanks for your gift to medicine, pain management and mankind. Your discovery of how to use these well researched reflexes to relieve pain is nothing short of transformational for both patients and practitioner alike. "

John R. Baird, MD. Louisville, KY

Chapter 8

Israeli Acupuncturist gets extraordinary results with PNT in an unbelievable number of conditions

Ran Kalif, LAc is an acupuncturist in Tel Aviv, Israel. As a practitioner of Traditional Chinese Medicine through acupuncture, the same as for general medical practitioners, he is exposed to a wide range of patients and pathologies. Mr. Kalif acquired PNT knowledge and experience and after a year of integrating this discipline to his practice then reported to Dr. Kaufman as follows:

"I've run a very busy practice in Tel Aviv, Israel for 25 years. Though I'm very successful and have had a heavily overbooked working schedule for many years, I do constantly look for new methods that work - to help my patients. I run a general practice and treat internal diseases, general neurology and orthopedics, GYN/fertility and also take endocrine cases.

*I've now been practicing the PNT techniques for a year. I took the time to really go deeply into the techniques, apply them efficiently, and use them extensively on the majority of my patients. Now that I have used the techniques on a **tremendous number of patients with a diversity of ailments** I can tell they're absolutely revolutionary. In many cases PNT puts some good techniques I have used before in the shade, both in terms of simplicity and efficacy, to the point I have abandoned them completely in favor of PNT and its various aspects. Here are some examples taken from hundreds of cases I've used PNT methods on:*

An 85 y/o male with 50 years frozen shoulder (his shoulder problem equals my age...) treated with PNT, the PNT Cervical Protocol and joint repositioning. He has regained full range of motion in less than a month (he shows up only once a week). His daughter sent him to me though he didn't believe it's even possible to gain relief after half a century of suffering. To tell you the truth, at first, neither did I.

A 60 y/o male underwent a medial meniscus surgery, following which he remained disabled to the point he could not fully flex and extend his knee. Walking without a stick wasn't even an option. After many months of unsuccessful rehabs and seeing many knee ortho specialists, he came to see me without any expectations. Now, after less than 3 months, he has returned to play tennis and even won 2 national senior contests, not to mention that he doesn't use a stick anymore and walks about completely normally.

A 50 y/o woman with an 18 month frozen shoulder with less than 30 degrees abduction ROM, no internal or external rotation ROM and less than 40 degrees extension ROM. She came with her husband with a thick medical documents file, after seeing numerous shoulder specialists and attending several rehab clinics. I learned from them that this issue has completely turned their life upside down. It will sound pretentious but it's the absolute truth to say, that after applying the joint repositioning on her, she has regained full ROM both abducting and extending her shoulder, while regaining almost 50% in lateral and internal rotation- and that is after less than 10 minutes when she first entered the treatment room. She looked at her husband and they both started to cry, hugging each other. My assistants, some are with me more than 15 years, couldn't believe their eyes. And so did I..., she came for a few more short sessions after which she returned to a normal life routine.

A 45 y/o medical doctor with a severe TMJ syndrome, which started after a shelf dropped on her head. Though she went to see several specialists, she gained no relief. She came for 5 sessions and I applied your cervical and TMJ treatments. She recovered completely, regaining full jaw ROM, stopped clenching during sleep, and felt no pain during the day.

A 25 y/o woman with severe vertigo to the point she couldn't walk alone down the street, making her totally debilitated in her daily routine. She went to see several neurologists and had CT, MRI and some more tests including hospitalization in a private medical facility. No pathology could be defined. After about 7 sessions utilizing the cervical and the vertigo procedures, she is almost symptom free.

A 58 y/o male suffering from excruciating LLQ abdominal pain that led him to the emergency room many times. After several colonoscopies and some more tests he was diagnosed as a diverticulitis case and was referred to a GI surgeon. When he first showed up at my clinic he could barely walk straight as the pain was too strong to bear. After less than 15 minutes, using your manual spinal nerve block procedures, he has regained complete relief. I have treated him several more times, though his pains never returned after the first session. Later on he called to report that his GI specialist said he is not a candidate for surgery anymore.

A 65 y/o woman with severe, chronic right arm radicular pain and thumb numbness. She came twice a week for about 6 weeks. I treated her with the cervical protocol and applied PNT on her upper back and neck. She's had total recovery from both pain and numbness.

A 45 y/o psychologist presented with chronic daily headaches dating back to her mid-twenties. Some are to the point of a debilitating migraine, shutting her down for three days. I have taught her spouse the occipital lift procedure, to be applied on her 3-4 minutes every other day. She had a complete recovery. I've known this woman for a long time now, and I can surely say it simply cured her headaches.

A 75 y/o woman suffering from a chronic toothache. After seeing several dentists, she was finally advised to have a root canal procedure. She was referred to me by one of my assistants, who knew my work. I applied the "rub lite" technique on her and taught one of her family member the trick, to be performed on her 3-4 times more. She called to report that her toothaches no longer exist and now after several months, it never returned to bother her.

A 38 y/o woman in her 36th week of pregnancy presented with a fetus in breech position. Her OB/GYN doctor told her she will need a cesarean, because he tried to perform physical flip under US scanning and couldn't make it. I treated her with PNT The next day she called to report that soon after leaving my clinic she felt a movement inside her, so she rushed to the doctor's office to perform a US scanning which showed her fetus now in a normal position. Later on she naturally delivered a healthy baby.

A 70 y/o woman with chest/rib trauma and unbearable pain gained no relief from pain pills and injections. When she first came in she could barely breathe, let alone laugh or sneeze without severe bouts of sharp pain. I used PNT on her including the rib technique, the Manual Spinal Nerve Block and the Sclerotome Techniques. After 20 minutes she walked out pain free to the amazement of both her husband and myself.

A 30 y/o man presented with multiple abdominal surgeries following acute intestinal blocks due to diverticular formations. When he came he presented these same acute pains previously leading him to the surgeon's operating room. I applied the manual spinal nerve block and the sclerotome techniques. When he came to see me two days later, he reported that soon after he left my clinic the first time, the pains subsided to the point he can hardly feel it. He was so happy to say that its the first time he can recall not ending with another abdominal surgery.

A 70 y/o male presenting with chest oppression, shortness of breath and weakness. All these symptoms started after open heart surgery a few years ago. I applied the diaphragm reflex and the sclerotome techniques for about 5 sessions. He gained complete recovery from the afore mentioned symptoms, allowing him to return to his previous job and walk freely without any breathing difficultly, just as he did prior to the heart surgery.

A 65 y/o male with post trauma tail bone pains, leaving him unable to sit and lay down in most positions. He went to several pain clinics but gained no relief. I saw him only twice, applying PNT on sacral trigger points and using the Gracilis Reflex Technique. He recovered completely and was actually able to sit after the first session.

I have many more, too many to count. Though I have gained much proficiency using the PNT techniques due to my busy practice and large volume of patients flow, I am still quite amazed by both its simplicity and astonishing efficacy."

Ran Kalif, LAc. Tel Aviv, Israel

Chapter 9

Pain Neutralization Technique

Practitioner's general reports

What follow are general testimonials from diverse practitioners which illustrate different aspects of PNT These, the same as all other testimonials are printed here largely unedited as they were sent to Dr. Kaufman. Of these general reports some carry redundant comments, yet all bring at least one description to help complete the picture of what PNT is about, and are worth reading.

*"**Here's a miracle I wouldn't have believed if I wasn't there to witness it**. A previously unknown chiropractor delivered a talk about his Pain Neutralization Technique for instantly relieving the pain of trigger points. He claimed to immediately restore motion and eliminate pain. What medical doctor would believe such claims from a chiropractor? I listened with curiosity and healthy skepticism. Then he performed his technique on many of my esteemed colleagues including some very famous ones. The majority got immediate relief, even with very long term chronic problems. It was absolutely incredible! I'll be devoting an issue of my newsletter to his techniques."*
Robert J. Rowen, MD editor-in- chief, "Second Opinion" newsletter. Santa Rosa, CA. May, 2006

*"Stephen is a miracle worker! I've had many different types of body work and chiropractic, but what he does is beyond anything else I've experienced. He **literally removes the cause of structural pain, and the pain stays gone!** I met him several yrs ago, have been fortunate enough to experience his work direct from him on several occasions, and I am always amazed and gratified.*

He's got the goods! I recommend that his seminar and DVDs be seen by every healer—body worker, DC, or other physician, and be the standard of care. Simply - it works. He's also an excellent teacher. It's one thing to be a master of your craft, and another to be able to convey it successfully to others. He does it all."
Hyla Cass, MD Bestselling author, Los Angeles, CA

"When Dr. Kaufman applied the technique the relief was so immediate I had to wait a few moments and focus on the spot to be certain I was feeling what I was feeling--or what I was not feeling any longer, if you get my meaning. A series of sports injuries and auto accidents beginning at age 7 have left me, at age 56, with daily bouts of neck pain, limited range of motion and inability to hold my head in one position for any length of time. Years of adjustments, acupuncture, massage and yoga brought only temporary relief. **Dr. Kaufman's treatment resulted in almost instant relief of muscle pain and normal, full range of motion.** *Many thanks for an exciting new and very effective modality."*
Bob Ratzow, DC Portland, OR

"After the conference I treated my patient's knees. She's now **sleeping pain free for the first time since last spring.** *Dr. K. also treated a patient yesterday for plantar fasciitis, a condition that has caused her considerable pain for about six months. Today she has no pain at all."*
Terry Chappell, MD, president, International College of Integrative Medicine, past president American College for Advancement in Medicine. Bluffton, OH

"I've had upper abdominal pain for one year, getting worse. After treatment by Dr. Kaufman, the pain on the left side went away, leaving the right side (not treated) feeling left out. On the break, I had a new practitioner work on the right side and got immediate relief. **It was amazing a new practitioner could get the same results!** *It's so easy! I'm amazed."*
Frank Alamilla, DC Ft Worth, TX

"I've had **chronic low back pain,** *SI [sacroiliac] joint pain for over a year. At times I had severe lumbar muscle spasms so in-*

tense I could barely walk. Dr. Kaufman, utilizing the Pain Control Points, **reduced my pain level by 80% immediately**, *and greatly improved my lumbar mobility. To have significant change in a matter of minutes was AMAZING!"*
Stanley Brown, PT. Springfield, MO

"I've had **chronic C5-6 pain** *since my mare dumped me in the pasture on my head* **50 years** *ago. At the ACAM meeting in Phoenix, 2007, the pain was relieved 90% that day and has remained so* **for over 6 months.** *At the Denver Boot Camp, I had chronic medial epicondylitis of the right elbow relieved by treatment."*
George R. Watson, D.O. Wichita, KS

"I came to the seminar as a 'respectful skeptic' but nothing could have prepared me for the unbelievable results I observed. *Problems that either respond slowly (or not all) in my office were eliminated in no time. This information will enhance my clinical skills immeasurably. As an added bonus, the constant upper trapezius pain I walked around with on a daily basis was greatly relieved right away. I feel very confident that I will be able to apply these procedures in my practice Monday morning."*
Michael Clancey, DC Fairmont, MN

"I can remember several years ago hearing about Pain Neutralization Technique and thinking to myself there was nothing to it. ***How could something so simple be effective in treating pain?*** *I waited 2 years and decided to look more closely at your website. Once I started reading I found myself unable to stop. The website is very compelling to read and the number of testimonials is unreal.* ***I ordered the basic PNT DVDs and could not be more amazed with the results I am getting with patients.*** *I took your advice and didn't change any of my treatments but simply added PNT* ***I've used PNT on over 100 patients with successful outcomes in all cases except one."***
Jay E. Young, DC Easley, SC

*"**I get so many compliments** (from PNT), it's unbelievable. PNT is brilliant. I can feel the trigger points dissolve under my fin-*

*gers. I had a guy walk in on crutches and walk out without them. I treated a 35 y/o female, who had chiropractic care, P.T., and a lumbar MRI. She had 3 lumbar spinal injections, which increased her pain. **After 2 weeks of PNT the patient is now working full time, after 3 months of disability**. Another 55 year old female had a lumbar fusion 5 years ago and had received spinal injections twice a year. PNT was more effective and lasted longer."*

Elliot J. Rampulla, MD Diplomate, American Board of Anesthesiology, American Academy of Pain Management, Former Assistant Professor of Anesthesiology and Pain Management at University of South Alabama College of Medicine

*"I've had pain/dysfunction in my right wrist for over a year and a half. I was pessimistic, having had many different musculoskeletal treatments for this, which were unsuccessful. However, with **one treatment with Dr. Kaufman's PNT my pain has gone and my wrist is back to functioning normally**. I've not been able to do a pushup for 18 months, and now I can. Many thanks. I cannot speak or recommend more highly this technique."*

Theo Peters MD, D.O., Diplomate, British Medical Acupuncture Society, Specialist National Health Service Consultant in Musculoskeletal Medicine at the Royal London Hospital for Integrated Medicine. MSK Specialist, Primary Care Rheumatology Society. Arundel, England

*"**I have been using Dr. Kaufman's techniques for 5+ years. I see amazing results every day**. Three weeks ago I had a 19 year old female come in 16 weeks pregnant. She had 10/10 pain from the low back down both legs with intermittent numbness and loss of bowel and bladder function. She was catheterized for 3 days and had not had a bowel movement in 7 days. My first impression was **Cauda Equina syndrome** so I sent her and her father to the E.R. They did an M.R.I. to rule out herniated disc and they returned for treatment. I neutralized many trigger points in her abdomen and pelvis/gluteals and legs. After **4 treatments her pain was completely resolved**. She was having bowel movements and her catheter was removed and she was able to urinate normally. I have found over and over that when you release pain*

you allow the body to stop its physiologic response to pain, and that's when the real miracles happen. Thanks again, Dr. Kaufman for changing my life and the lives of my patients."
Reuben Mickel, DC Vancouver, WA

"Wow! That's amazing! **Dr Kaufman worked on my right psoas and right low back and the pain, discomfort, and guarding I have had for the past month** *– since I sprained my back –* **was gone – completely gone!** *It no longer feels like if I make one wrong move that it will "go out" again. This is unbelievably wonderful. There are a couple of things I'd like to say about PNT: first, sometimes we see a teacher do amazing things to help people, but we are not really able to duplicate his work. Well,* **with PNT and the way Dr. Kaufman teaches and the DVD's this work is absolutely duplicable.** *The second point is* **PNT is off of the power grid, in terms of healing techniques!"**
P.J. Zaramskas, LAc. Pollock Pines, CA

"Many people are hard wired in their brain to believe only what they believe, which is most of the time what everyone else is saying. By using Dr Kaufman's techniques the results are both immediate and measurable in my gym. Muscles, because of poor reflexes/motor patterns fight against one another instead of working with each other in concert to provide a desired movement. This is called a compensation pattern and it results in inhibition or a lack of ability to readily activate a motor unit. Because the human body is so wonderful, it figures out how to move with these patterns any ways. The unfortunate part is we tend to then strengthen these patterns in regular training and reinforce them during games. This leads to injury, stalled training, or over-training.
The key to strength and speed training is eliminating these patterns; return the athlete to the correct movement pattern, then strengthen and increase their ability to absorb force. With these simple techniques that I implement from Dr. Kaufman, we can change the compensatory movement pattern and get immediate responses in training. These immediate responses include but are not limited to increased strength, mobility, recovery time, lowering of heart rate, and reversal of poor firing patterns. This

has taken my training protocols to a new level!!! I have put 2 inches on an athlete's vertical jump using the Paradoxical muscle reflex. I have changed the foot strike position in sprinting using the gird technique. I have increased someone's bench press by 3 reps using the Meridian Bending techniques. The accolades and superlatives are endless because I use it every day as a performance tool. It's what separates me from the ordinary strength trainers.

I hope to work closely with Dr. Kaufman on future endeavors in an untapped field. Results are visible, new standards are being set, and you are going to wonder why you didn't learn about these techniques earlier."
Dan Fichter, Owner Wannagetfast.com Pittsford, NY

"Following the PNT class in June of 2010 I returned to my Physical Therapy practice where I treated 17 patients and had incredible results with turning off all pain in 15 of the 17 patients. This has been the best technique I've ever learned in my 30 years of PT practice. My patients are in awe of it. Thanks Steve so much for sharing these techniques with us."
Teena Petree, PT. Plano, TX

"I'm still performing the PNT techniques with very good success (2 years after the boot camp). ***My practice only uses your techniques.****"*
Marvin H Wilson, MD, Vascular Surgeon. Topeka, KS

"The Pain Elimination Boot Camp last year was ***the best thing that I've done educationally in 30 years of practice****."*
Debbie Powell, PT. Jackson, AL

"Dr. Kaufman is a ***true innovator****. He has a wide variety of brilliant techniques that produce real and rapid results. While he may not have evidence-based studies due to the newness of his techniques, he produces evidence-based results in real time—often in seconds."*
Todd Pollock, PT. Kasilof, AK

"2 weeks after I attended the June 2010 Boot Camp, I held a seminar, partly to introduce the techniques I learned from Dr. Kaufman. I bravely decided to take my chances by asking for volunteers from the audience to see if I could relieve their pain from tender trigger points. A dozen people volunteered to put me on the spot. **To my amazement, to the patients' amazement, to the audience's amazement, every person who volunteered reported complete relief of tenderness after less than a minute of treatment.** *I don't expect 100% effectiveness in the future, but I trust these treatments to melt away my patients' trigger points and substantially improve the quality of their lives."*
Terry Chappell, MD, president, International College of Integrative Medicine, past president American College for Advancement in Medicine. Bluffton, OH

"I had one patient with severe bone pain from melanoma- gone, after treatment. Many, many others with severe, chronic pain-gone! **Not only were the results on other patients/physicians stunning, but also the treatment I had: in 2-3 seconds, all of my own trigger points and facet pain disappeared!** *"It's amazing!" and* **"It's gone!"** *are exactly what I hear from my own patients: it's a hoot! Your techniques have* **added a HUGE new dimension to my practice**; *they put the fun back in, after 43 years."*
David Walsh MD, Pain Management Specialist, Diplomat, American Board of Pain Medicine; Diplomat, American Board of Anesthesiology. Mobile, AL

"A while back I ordered the basic PNT DVDs + cervical combo. I started watching them over a weekend and within the first hour pretty much grokked what to do. Presently I work in PI so nearly everything I see is MVA related. I decided to roll out my new PNT skills to a select few of my patients to see how well I could make it work. It's worth mentioning that most of my patients speak a language other than my native tongue and communication is somewhat sketchy. So I picked patients with just enough English to understand questions like "Is that a sore spot?" and "Does that make it better?"
In 15 years I have never been compelled to write a testimonial about a "technique" before. So if you think this is lengthy and

that I'm verbose it's only in direct proportion to my amazement about how EASY this is and how EFFECTIVE it is. I was pretty good at what I did before and have been exposed to a good smattering of stuff across the chiropractic spectrum, from the classic to the esoteric. And I have NEVER seen anything work like this. This is not hyperbole to say that in the first few weeks (1) I had become a better doctor by an exponential degree, (2) I felt a bonding with the people on my table that I didn't feel before and (3) I became happier practicing than I had been in a long, long time. I'm reliving the same feelings many of us had when we came out of school ready to fix everybody and still naïvely thinking that all the stuff we were taught would work just like they said it would. A few years in practice beat down some of that enthusiasm. But if chiropractic schools taught PNT as the treatment gold-standard (along with better nutritional and functional medicine training, IMO) and dumped a lot of the other "technique" stuff they promulgate I truly believe that outside of surgical emergencies and a few other things we could be the dominant health profession on earth.

Incidentally I think calling PNT or Kaufman Technique a "technique" is minimizing what it is. It is true that it contains a variety of techniques but it is a MODEL. It has become a trite phrase but PNT is truly a "paradigm shift". It is, in my opinion, a fundamentally different way of approaching a human being with pain or other health problems than anything else out there. It's bigger than just another "technique". I for one never gave trigger points their due as the nasty little termites they are, much less thought about ever "turning them off". I think that your triceps extension experience was an Isaac Newton moment in its magnitude. And I mean that sincerely. To any interested parties, I have never met Dr. Kaufman and I've only watched DVDs and then only those on the basic PNT level (no Manual Spinal Nerve Blocks or Grid Patterns or Pain Control Patterns or any of that stuff. I don't even know what any of that is – but I plan to. My conclusion after working with these procedures is that everything on Dr. Kaufman's website is absolutely true."

Ross Vaughn, DC, DACACD(c). Longwood, FL

*"Had I not seen it, I wouldn't have believed a system based on simple body physiology could take away your pain so quickly. I and 40 other doctors witnessed several dozen consecutive resolutions or near total relief of chronic pain. Dr. Kaufman's remarkable technique might resolve your chronic pain or even organ dysfunction. **It's so simple it's astonishing the technique is unknown in medical school and largely unknown even to chiropractors**. If you're like the dozens of physicians I witnessed, you'll exclaim, "wow, that's amazing", or "I just can't believe it." Here's a "hands on" technique that heals the multitudes, by resetting their nervous system reflexes."*

Robert J. Rowen, MD editor-in- chief, "Second Opinion" newsletter. Santa Rosa, CA

Chapter 10

PNT Cases: Specific Reports

The following sections include reports Dr. Kaufman received by the time this book was being finished. The reports are organized by areas of the body, loosely grouping them in distinct syndromes for each area. This reporting is **intended** to serve **as a general guide** for the **reader to** be able to **correlate** his or her **own personal experience with the experience of practitioners and patients** collected thus far. Also this reporting does not intend by any means to be an all-inclusive listing of what PNT can accomplish. In these reports the reader may find occasional apparent discrepancies in the terminologies (labels) used to describe the different syndromes. Because these reports cross over the boundaries of many healthcare disciplines these occasional and apparent discrepancies are inevitable.

While the way human biology works in general is one —with many subtle individual variables, the way **each individual discipline** got started and developed is particular to each. This individuality, at least in part, relates to the **limited perspective of the whole t**aken by each one given discipline and its creator/developer, and to the fact that in general terms each discipline evolved **with some degree of isolation from the others**.

On the other hand it can be useful for the reader to keep in mind that these boundaries between disciplines are as real to Medicine as the lines drawn in a map to delineate countries are to Mother Earth. **Medicine and health care are** in essence **about people with health problems and about information and ways to** more or less effectively **resolve them**; nothing more. The **boundaries between disciplines are not real**; they are inevitable constructs emerging as a consequence of the way we human beings set out to do things, our purposes, intentions, and "rules of engagement."

What follows is an index broadly organizing the reports by body area and for each area, by individual syndromes. The last section includes syndromes that are more generalized, more systemic or functional for lack of a better and simpler terminology. The interested reader can then refer to any particular series of reports of interest using this index or enjoy the wide variety of experiences -in many instances most remarkable- included herein.

It goes without saying that the PNT techniques do not work on every patient. Not every patient or every condition responds to PNT Some patients respond partially or do not respond at all. Several treatments are usually needed for lasting results. The following reports are some of our best cases as doctors have reported them; they have not been verified by the authors. No particular result can be guaranteed on any patient, and the authors are not responsible for the outcome, positive or negative, of treatment by any practitioner using these techniques. Calculating generally expected performance results is difficult or impossible, because there is no "typical" patient or doctor. We've made a good faith effort to share the actual experiences of our practitioners and their patients.

Indexed specific reports

Chapter 11
Head and Neck

Headaches

"A patient wrote me the following testimonial: "I've had severe neck pain and headaches since an auto accident in 1986; I had 3 fractures at C4, C5 and C6. I have tried every kind of medical and alternative treatment I could find. I walked into Dr. Salas' office July 18 at 10:00 A.M., and walked out at 11:00 A.M. without a headache! It's 4 weeks since this treatment and I'm still free of the headache that has plagued me for almost twenty years."
Alain Salas, DC Kansas City, MO

"I had dramatic results getting rid of excruciating posterior head and neck pain using the Mandibular Reflex in a 71-year old male patient with post-shingles pain. I also used the Sclerotome Technique to help a 58-year old female with a tender lateral atlas and a pounding headache. Relief was immediate in both cases, and to the best of my knowledge, lasting."
Stuart Marmorstein, DC Houston, TX

"I bought the PNT DVD's and have been getting consistently good results with my patients. Recently I treated a lady who was getting constant headaches, and had to take a lot of pain medication to get through the day; within three visits (with PNT) she had no more headaches."
Suhill Samji, DC Vancouver, British Columbia, Canada

"I just had a patient who had severe headache and neck pain for 20 years with neck range of motion limited to only 20° on the left. He has been to every possible physician and chiropractor known to him in the last 5 years. PNT meridian Bending caused his neck pain and headache to go away instantly with complete active ROM, without any assisting. The guy left in surprise and happy, which made me happy. Please note he was here for his narcotic

medication and was crying in pain before this procedure. Amazing..."
Jawad Bhatti, MD   Midlothian, VA

"I've had severe neck pain and severe occipital headaches for 15 years. The neck pain was constant, the headaches 40% of the time. I searched desperately for an answer through numerous chiropractic techniques with very little response. At the bootcamp I quickly had 65-70% reduction of pain and a very distinct increase in my ROM. 36 hours later that relief is still the same. I haven't had lasting relief like this in over a decade."
David E. Fray, DC Raytown, MO

"Since an auto accident in 1982 I've had cervical discomfort, loss of ROM and sub-occipital headaches. After Dr. Kaufman treated me yesterday about 90% of the pain in the lower C-spine was removed. The ROM is near normal, upper c-spine pain is still gone and I have no sub-occipital or frontal region headache. Much of this pain has been with me for over 26 years!"
Robert McCartney, DC Chouteau, OK

"I had a lady come in with severe headaches and hip pain after a fall almost a year ago. She has been walking with a cane since the fall. She came in a day after the first treatment and was walking without a cane. I have seen her a few times since and she states that the hip pain is almost totally gone, except for going up or down stairs which still bothers her a little but is continuing to improve. Her headaches have not returned since the second visit.
"A lady came in with severe headaches and tingling in the temporal region. She also had low back pain. Her complaints were so severe she had to close her clothing store. The Sclerotome Techniques™ and PNT resolved the headaches, the tingling in her head and her low back pain. She is now in the process of opening up another clothing store."
Terry Williams, DC Ft. Lupton, CO

"Wow" doesn't begin to cover the relief I feel (after PNT treatment)! I was diagnosed with Arnold Chiari Malformation and had decompression surgery in 2002. 4 years later, I had 2 cervical disc

surgeries. Though the more serious neurological symptoms are controlled, I've had daily headaches, neck stiffness, and chronic cervical pain since then. Regular physical therapy, deep tissue massage, and medication helped somewhat, but any relief was temporary. One treatment (with the PNT techniques) has relieved the painful stiffness and limited range of motion of the past 10 years!! My father (also a physician) had hopes of a small miracle (from PNT) MISSION ACCOMPLISHED! My family medicine practice has <u>many</u> chronic pain patients. I hope I can afford them even a fraction of the relief I feel from the PNT techniques."
Rhodora Kabatay- Lee Ho, MD Pekin, IL

Migraines

"Since the seminar in June 2010, I've had much success in treating chronic ITB syndrome, lumbar pain, SI dysfunction and upper trapezius myofascial pain. Acute migraines have substantially decreased on the spot! Kaufman Techniques are a wonderful addition to my acupuncture/osteopathic practice, gentle, non-invasive...and effective!"
Rosalie Bondi, D.O. Arvada, CO

"A 45 y/o psychologist presented with chronic daily headaches dating back to her mid-twenties. Some are to the point of a debilitating migraine, shutting her down for three days. I have taught her spouse the occipital lift procedure, to be applied on her 3-4 minutes every other day. She had a complete recovery. I've known this woman for a long time now, and I can surely say it simply cured her headaches."
Ran Kalif, LAc. Tel Aviv, Israel

"I wanted to send a little report regarding using the PNT Techniques. I remember reporting to you that I could sometimes perceive a palpable release or pulsation at trigger points as I applied PNT And I thought that was way cool. Still do. But that in no way compares to the dramatic pulsating release that both I and my patient felt as I as I did the PNT Technique Reflex™ to release an occipital trigger point. My patient responded with "WHAT THE

HECK WAS THAT!?" I was treating her for migraine headache which included hypersensitivity of most all of her scalp to the lightest of touch. Following the palpable occipital release, the migraine was gone, the scalp hypersensitivity was gone, and I am once again in awe of this material. Thank you so much."
Marcus Smith, M.S., AP.   Coral Springs, FL

"Recently, I treated a lady who had been injured in an auto accident. She had pain throughout her body, and mostly was experiencing migraine headaches. The migraine headaches and body pain were onboard twenty-fours hours a day. All of this had been going on for one month. She was bedridden several hours each day and hadn't been able to work. She is a young mother of three children. Previous to when I saw her, she was under the care of an MD and a chiropractor. I spent about six minutes using only PNT When she got up from the table, her face had a huge smile. Her body pain and more importantly to her the migraine headache was gone – completely! I treated her ONCE! WOW!"
Fred Eckfeld, DC Santa Barbara, CA

TMJ syndrome, jaw clicking, teeth grinding

*"I had suffered with TMJ for many years that came with a loud clicking sound, which was seriously annoyed my husband. One treatment with Dr. Kaufman permanently resolved the issue. **The click and the palpatory tenderness cleared up immediately, and the jaw healed itself completely over the next few months.** I am happy to say that I have completely recovered and no longer consider myself to have a TMJ issue."*
Lisa Howie, LMT. Aspen, CO

*"My 14 year-old son, Allen, had a 'popping' jaw, causing him a lot of discomfort. **After a very brief treatment the 'popping' was gone!** Very impressive results!! **2 week follow up: the jaw has not clicked at all since the seminar."***
Curt Maxwell, MD Yuma, AZ

"A 45 y/o medical doctor with a severe TMJ syndrome, which started after a shelf dropped on her head. Though she went to see several specialists, she gained no relief. She came for 5 sessions and I applied your cervical and TMJ treatments. She recovered completely, regaining full jaw ROM, stopped clenching during sleep, and felt no pain during the day."
Ran Kalif, LAc. Tel Aviv, Israel

"I've had jaw pain (TMJ) for over 30 years. 2 broken jaws (mandible fractures) 2 surgeries, 3+ months of the denture and still lots of pain. After 2 minutes of treatment, my TMJ feels 50% better!"
Stephen Irestone, DC   Burnsville, MN

"By applying Dr. Kaufman's revolutionary techniques, TMJ treatments became much easier and faster. Patients love it so much, and I am enjoying my TMJ practice without tension or stress. I had 42-year-old lady with clicking and popping jaw; it became quiet in a minute using Dr. Kaufman's technique. The very limited mouth opening (38mm) also went up to 45 mm instantly. A 26-year-old lady had migraine and neck aches, related to her TMJ; they were relieved after only one session. She also reported that her facial asymmetry has been improving."
Sang Duk Lee, D.D.S. Beverly Hills, CA

"I have been suffering from major accidents, the first a car accident in 2003, and second in 2009, and 2 other serious falls. I had 3 concussions in the last 11 years and daily life has been very difficult. I avoid moving and my neck that has been significantly painful and when I do move my neck, it has been most limited. And I always avoid forward flexion and extension- my range of motion for my waist and my neck are at about 30 degrees. After Dr. Kaufman's PNT magic I had up to 90 degrees. That is amazing! My neurologist implied that my condition was probably permanent as I was not responding to various modalities of physical therapy treatments. My last TMJ exam with the specialist said to me that I needed a 6 year treatment plan that included several surgeries, orthodontics for 4 years, and other treatments including several years of different splints. After this extensive plan, the specialist

said I still may have the pain, but at least I'd be able to open my mouth to eat. For years I have had to either puree or dice my foods in order to eat. All chewing, even cottage cheese, is painful.

Dr Kaufman treated my TMJ. At the break following my treatment, I stopped in my room to freshen up. To my astonishment and amazement, while washing my teeth, I stopped in my tracks, realizing in the first time in 5 to 6 years I was brushing my molars. My mouth could open to actually get my toothbrush over my molars to brush them. In years I have only been able to get a water pick to my molars for cleaning. Even my hygienist can't complete her cleaning and my dentist of 25 years has referred me out because he can't get an instrument in my mouth. Also, incredibly, I brushed my hair, being able to push my neck in a forward flexion position. Wow! Most importantly, I didn't get the twinkle lights that I get when putting my head forward, down, or in that forward flexion movement. Also, I had soup and salad for dinner and didn't need to chop up the lettuce into itsy bitsy ½ inch pieces. After chewing, my jaw wasn't sore. Today, again, my toothbrush fit in my mouth and amazingly, I could even floss for the first time all of my teeth easily (first time in 5 years). My hygienist never can do any flossing during my cleaning. My mouth can open with at least 2 fingers spread now without pain and yesterday before PNT treatment I couldn't put even one finger in my mouth. This morning I even washed my hair, raising my arms over my head without getting dizzy or seeing twinkle lights. Also, I'm still amazed that I can turn my head side to side without having to turn my body. I didn't even use my hand splint last night and my jaw felt relaxed this morning. I've been wearing splints since my first car accident in 2003.

I am most grateful to Dr. Kaufman for sharing his talents and giftedness that has freed my jaw and neck from severe pain and serious restrictions. Also, another doctor attending this seminar for PNT said he thought I looked 15 years younger after my treatment. Wow! Thank you Dr. Kaufman, this is better and easier than plastic surgery. Looks like PNT is also great for anti-aging. That's an amazing bonus!"

Donna Phelps (Wife of Ron Phelps, DC) Mission Viejo, CA

"After 5 years of TMJ pain, Dr. Kaufman demonstrated a 3 minute treatment on me. I am amazed how great I feel!"
Christian Distefano, LAc. Suffern, NY

Vision problems

"Also this from one of my patients: "During the past 4 years I've had vision problems in my left eye. As time went on my vision got worse with greater impairment. I saw a neurologist. Eventually I found myself nearly unable to function as a police officer as my vision in my left eye was now impaired 24/7. In June of 2008 I went to Dr. Raether in desperation. With his techniques I've experienced relief in the first week. Within 4 weeks the symptoms were gone and stayed away. My vision is completely restored and I have Dr Raether to thank for that."
Charles Raether, DC New Holstein, WI

"I've had 2 years of cervical pain that often radiates to the right rhomboid and up the right side of head. After 2 minutes of the cervical protocol, the pain is gone! A side effect of that is clearer vision (was foggy before treatment) and rising energy."
Yonat Harnov, AP. Coral Springs, FL

"There have been quite a few cases of poor eyesight improvement demonstrated by the need to change prescriptions for the better."
Mark Sinclair, DC Auckland, New Zealand

Vertigo – Dizziness - Tinnitus (ringing in the ear) – Hearing loss

"Recently a lady with a history of migraine that I have been treating with acupuncture/moxa and Chinese herbal medicine hit her head hard enough for a mild concussion, which stimulated a rocking side to side vertigo as well as headache. She did not complain of tinnitus. I used the posterior auricular tendon twist and her vertigo stopped within 10 seconds, I went on to neutralize her tender points, which were the SCM attachment at the mastoids, and her

left levator scapulae at SI 13. The occipital lift made her feel worse, but the cervical stairstep made her feel better. She was agitated and fearful so I thought I would try the inferior cervical sympathetic ganglion, but she hated this. I did the forehead squash instead. She left feeling almost normal."
Lee Grotte, MD Cleveland, OH

"Two separate cases of severe vertigo, both having been hospitalized for a few days, one having constant vomiting, (arrived with a bucket), the other having had the dizziness accompanied by visual disturbances. Both received treatment sitting, following the vertigo protocol on the sagittal plane only. Both treatments took only 3-4 minutes. Follow-up visit a few days later in each case found 90% improvement. 100% improvement took a few more visits while dealing with other issues."
Mark Sinclair, DC Auckland, New Zealand

"A 25 y/o woman with severe vertigo to the point she couldn't walk alone down the street, making her totally debilitated in her daily routine. She went to see several neurologists and had CT, MRI and some more tests including hospitalization in a private medical facility. No pathology could be defined. After about 7 sessions utilizing the cervical and the vertigo procedures, she is almost symptom free."
Ran Kalif, LAc. Tel Aviv, Israel

"The Kaufman Vertigo protocol has been a godsend. I took a gentleman with 30+ years of vertigo to the point of being asymptomatic in 1 treatment. This gentleman would rise with vertigo every morning and would have to hold his head in his hands for 15 minutes before he could stand erect. Suffice to say he insists I perform the treatment on him monthly."
 Brent J. Mills, MSc., DC Kingston, Ontario, Canada

"Tinnitus is about as tough to treat problem as exists. It is about as much fun treating as having a tooth pulled. Yet on 2 occasions, using the mandibular-maxillary technique, the patients remarked on great improvement. That probably approaches my previous 30+ year total. Oh yes, the Mandibular reflex also alleviates most

trap pain, and just about every time. It puts in the hand of the drugless clinician, a potent weapon against head and neck problems that is disproportional to any effort extended."
Steven Lavitan, DC, LAc. former columnist, Dynamic Chiropractic. Paramus, NJ

"I've used the Mandibular Reflex on several patients with tinnitus, and seen substantial improvement in all of them. (I also have them treat the reflex daily for 20 seconds."
David Walsh MD, Pain Management Specialist, Diplomat, American Board of Pain Medicine; Diplomat, American Board of Anesthesiology. Mobile, AL

"A woman, 56 year old, lost her hearing after she caught a bad cold 2 months before. She saw a lot of ENT and neurological doctors with no result. I treated her with cervical and vertigo protocol. The second day she text me that she had over the night some popping sounds in her ears, but next morning her hearing came back."
Dr. Dacian Hulber, MD Bucharest, Romania

Other chronic head pains

"I saw a lady with severe oral pain for 3 years who had been to MANY doctors. She also had pain down the back of her neck to her elbow. I did the Mandibular Reflex bilaterally and all the pain in her mouth stopped. Her mouth went NUMB. In fact she felt pulsation in her tongue (indicating increased blood flow.) She actually left the office crying tears of joy."
David Walsh MD, Pain Management Specialist, diplomat, American Board of Pain Medicine; diplomat, American Board of Anesthesiology. Mobile, AL

"I had chronic suboccipital pain for about 5 years. Dr. Kaufman treated me and I am NOT experiencing any more pain in the suboccipitals and my range of movement has increased."
Timothy Smith, LMT. Hollywood, FL

"I treated a female, 45 years old. 18 years before she had tongue cancer spread into the lymph nodes. She had surgery and radiation

to treat the cancer. As a result of surgery, she was hypersensitive on right neck and side of her face to the point that she could not touch her neck or face for 18 years. I treated her with the Manual Spinal Nerve Block and her neck and face are now completely normal for the first time in 18 years. Her comment: 'Unbelievable, amazing.' She was referred to me by a local physician."
Martin Benjamin, LAc. Lenox, MA

Acute and chronic neck pain – Whiplash injury

"When Dr. Kaufman applied the technique the relief was so immediate I had to wait a few moments and focus on the spot to be certain of what I was feeling--or what I was not feeling any longer, if you get my meaning. Injuries and auto accidents from age 7 left me, at 56, with daily neck pain, limited range of motion and inability to hold my head in one position for any length of time. Years of adjustments, acupuncture, massage and yoga brought only temporary relief. Treatment resulted in almost instant relief of muscle pain and normal, full range of motion."
Bob Ratzow, DC Portland, OR

"I had a painful upper trapezius for several years following a chiropractic adjustment to my shoulder. The pain was gone with a treatment that took seconds, at the boot camp. My diaphragm then released and I could breathe easier! One night, I was awakened by my friend who was in pain and couldn't sleep, from pain following dental work. I was half awake, used two techniques, and it was gone!"
Aleae Pennette, DC Santa Rosa, CA

"I've been living with chronic neck, shoulder, trap, rhomboid pain for as long as I can remember. With treatment of less than 2 minutes Dr. Kaufman eliminated the neck and trap pain."
Kate Canfield, AP. New Smyrna Beach, FL

"I had a severe neck injury 10 years ago and re-injured with whip-lash months ago. Recently I've had bad rhomboid cramping. After PNT: I have no pain!"
Helen Watt, MD Cave Creek, AZ

"My neck has been hurting on and off for 30+ years. I was in 12 auto accidents between the ages of 18-20. I'm 52 and have had chronic problems resulting from the repeated whiplash injuries. I have 5 bulging discs and 1 herniated disc. I've experienced imme-diate relief from Dr. Kaufman's techniques, and profound relaxa-tion."
Jenny Thompson, MD Parma, MI

"I've suffered chronic neck and shoulder pain for 15 years, from various sports and car accident injuries. I usually have to get ag-gressive chiropractic adjustments in order to get relief. After just 2 minutes of treatment, I feel great!"
Tom Grant, DC Salt Lake City, Utah

"I've had neck pain for 25 years. I twisted my neck lifting a patient. I've tried all sorts of treatments, chiropractors, acupuncture, mas-sage, electromagnetic frequency, zero point wand, bio energy and Rolfing to name a few. But I still had pain on palpitation, stiffness and chronic tightness. I also had a tender spot coming from C6. During the Pain Elimination Techniques seminar I was treated by Dr. Kaufman and some of the participants. My neck pain and stiff-ness are almost gone with just a few treatments. It's fantastic stuff."
Aine Delaney, LAc. SRN Galway, Ireland

"Since a bicycle accident and subsequent treatment in 1985, I have had chronic upper trap/neck pain. Acupuncture helps, but I al-ways know it is there. In addition to pain, my rotation to the right has been limited. After my treatment with Dr. Kaufman this morn-ing, I no longer notice the pain in my trap! First time in 27 years. Amazing!"
Donna Broomfall Cain, LAc. Ridgefield, CT

"Dr. Kaufman also treated my chronic tenderness at C6-T2 last October (10/2011). Now, nine months later, I can still report improved motion and greatly reduced pain in that area. Wow! Now that's amazing."
Mark Seitz, DC Dayton, OH

"The mechanism of this treatment (PNT) made sense to me but experiencing the treatment was almost shocking. I had burning C6-7 pain for 3-4 months that resolved in seconds. Without pressure or coaxing. It just resolved. And it's still gone the next day, by the way."
Dorothy Pedtke, D.O. Grand Rapids, MI

"I have had pain in C5, 6, 7 and was on disability for 11 weeks due to weakness and aching pain to the right arm in 2012. I had physical therapy and it helped a little but in the past 6 months the pain has worsened. I was planning on retiring next year. Wade Baskin, P.T. did the cervical protocol and worked on trigger points in my back during the 2012 Pain Elimination Bootcamp. The pain is gone and I am able to rotate my head with a much greater range of motion."
Valerie O'Rouke, R.N. Elk Grove, CA

"Also, as soon as I got back to my clinic I used the new Sclerotome Techniques™ to neutralize my Physical Therapy Assistant student's tension and soreness in his upper trapezius muscles. He stated he has had pain in this area for the last 2 years . He immediately noted less tension in his shoulders, but about an hour later stated that he could not remember the last time he had no tension in his shoulder and neck regions. I only spent about 1 minute doing the procedure. He was so amazed he then used the Sclerotome Techniques to turn off trigger points in our volunteer's neck. He was so excited to be able to instantly help someone. He'd never seen this type of success before. The technique is quick and easy to learn and just as quick to provide relief. What I love about PNT is that I can now do in 5-10 minutes what used to take 4-5 treatments. The combination of Trigger point elimination with Joint Repositioning for shoulder conditions consistently gives me such

quick results that the patients are astounded, it seemed "too easy" to them."
Mark Milleville, PT. Wheatfield, NY

Limited neck rotation

"WOW-AMAZING! I love the expression you see when the patient feels the pain just disappear. I used the occipital lift on a patient with limited C-spine ROM and did in 1 minute what I was unable to do in 4 months: restore full ROM without pain. You should have seen the expression on her face! "
Rick L. Townsend, DC, NMD, LAc. St. Robert, MO

"Several trigger points and pain in my neck disappeared right away. My range of motion to the right was very limited. Now I can turn my head fully to the right without pain."
Deborah Laplante (Wife of Andre Laplante, DC) Gatineau, Quebec, Canada

"I've had neck pain and significant decreased ROM since '95. After one treatment I now have full ROM without pain and stiffness. Even my sinuses opened up and I realize how tense my face/scalp muscles were, which now feel fully relaxed."
Donna Guthery, LAc. Bellaire, TX

"I myself had neck pain and restricted motion especially to the left. Dr. Steve treated me and immediately rotation was restored. Amazing. I have treated many people, but this is the first time for myself. My neck problem is eighteen years of duration, accident caused when I hit cement center divider on freeway, going backwards. I had many types of treatment and years later, no results. I'm excited for future progress."
Fred Eckfeld, DC Santa Barbara, CA

Paresthesia, numbness and other cervical radiculopathies (signs of nerve root compression)

"A 65 y/o woman with severe, chronic right arm radicular pain and thumb numbness. She came twice a week for about 6 weeks. I treated her with the cervical protocol and applied PNT on her upper back and neck. She's had total recovery from both pain and numbness."
Ran Kalif, LAc. Tel Aviv, Israel

"Dr. Kaufman's techniques are amazing! I had chronic lumbar pain for 15 years, due to L5 disc thinning and erosion. I needed constant and frequent adjustments. After treatment, my pain has gone and my flexibility is greatly improved! Also for the past 10 years I had chronic pain and limited rotation in the cervical area, and numbness in my right arm. At the seminar, Dr. Kaufman restored 95% cervical rotation and eliminated the numbness in my arm."
Sorina Durante, CMT, CLT. Lakewood, NJ

"One woman in her late 70's having had paresthesia in her Left C5 dermatome for several years, noted that after the first adjustment with the cervical protocol, it vanished and has never returned. She continues to see improvement as she continues her care."
Mark Sinclair, DC Auckland, New Zealand

"I was in an auto accident 5 months ago which left me with bilateral hand pain, limited cervical ROM w/ pain, right shoulder pain, and constant pressure in my lower cervicals. After treatment I have no shoulder pain, increased ROM, very small amount of pressure on lower cervical spine and my hands feel improved. The pains I listed are the ones left over after 5 months of chiropractic treatment. 2 weeks ago a surgical consultation was recommended. After treatment today, I am 95% improved. Thermography also shows a huge improvement."
George Freeland, DC Sparta, MI

"35 y/o patient with T1 spinal cord injury who's paraplegic has a bullet lodged in his neck with cervical radiculopathy and forearm pain bilaterally. He had 80% relief from manual spinal nerve blocks."
Jawad Bhatti, MD Midlothian, VA

"I treated a bodybuilder whose left arm, hand and fingers were paralyzed, since fracturing 4 cervical vertebrae 2 years ago. He'd had surgery at that time and was in hospital for 8 weeks. He couldn't move his fingers. 40 doctors and neurologists had told him he would never regain use of his arm and hand. He had zero deep tendon reflexes in his triceps and biceps. His fingers, biceps and triceps were absolutely paralyzed. On the first visit, using meridian bending and other PNT techniques, he regained full strength in his arm muscles, and almost full movement in his fingers. All his deep tendon reflexes came back. Feeling returned to his hand. His hand had looked very pale; almost full color came back after treatment. Both he and his wife started crying; his wife continued to cry for 10 minutes. This patient was referred in by a young girl who'd had severe migraines for 8 years. Her migraines stopped after two PNT treatments."
Marcus Seuthe, DC Black Forest, Baierbsronn, Germany

Chapter 12

Chest

Thoracic pain

"I have a patient who had chronic, unrelenting upper thoracic pain for many years. She responded poorly and temporarily to many techniques. During one of her worst flares I used Dr. Kaufman's pain relief technique; it quickly gave her 95% relief. Truly amazing! After 30+years of practice, this is the first testimonial I've ever written!"
Perry Ruby, DC Denver, CO

"I've had thoracic burning pain for 38 years. It gets relieved by weekly adjustments but always returns within minutes. Today, after a PNT Sclerotome Treatment™, I had the most profound relief I've experienced. This includes better posture, relaxation, and easier breathing."
Steven Lavitan, DC, LAc. former columnist, Dynamic Chiropractic. Paramus, NJ

"I've had severe chronic thoracic spine pain for years. I get chiropractic manipulations, massage, intersegmental traction, even back rubs. Pain relief was always short lived from a few hours to a few days. Ever since my first seminar with you, 1 ½ years ago, the PNT used on my mid back has lasted all that time. Today there was only one spot that released in seconds and feels great now."
Bill Strempel, DC Denver, CO

Rib pain

"A 70 y/o woman with chest/rib trauma and unbearable pain gained no relief from pain pills and injections. When she first came

in she could barely breathe, let alone laugh or sneeze without a severe bouts of sharp pain. I used PNT on her including the rib technique, the Manual Spinal Nerve Block and the Sclerotome Techniques. After 20 minutes she walked out pain free to the amazement of both her husband and me."
Ran Kalif, LAc. Tel Aviv, Israel

"I had very painful ribs for 2 years, off and on. After a brief 2 minute Basic Paraspinal PNT — the pain turned off, <u>gone</u>! This was so simple. Amazing, thank you! I also worked on a massage therapist with chronic arm and hand and elbow issues, and achieved great relief for her."
Karyn Erickson, LMT. Malvern, FL

Shortness of breath – asthma – COPD

"With all the classes I've attended with Dr. Kaufman, I still learn incredibly useful new information in each class. The respiratory protocol has been very successful in helping people breathe. I've had right hip pain and knee pain nearly a year, limited, painful range of motion. Dr. Kaufman eliminated several trigger points in a very short time and the knee pain is gone, immediately. I've had a burning nerve pain in the right thumb on elbow and thumb extension. Dr. Kaufman eliminated the burning with a treatment that took less than one minute."
Kerry Randa, DC Loveland, CO

"I saw a 68 year old woman with an enlarged heart and difficulty breathing, with moderately severe pain (7/10) throughout the thoracic and cervical spine. She's had pain for 8 years, constant for the last 6 months. She has had all manner of testing and paid $10,000 cash out of her pocket to get some answers. These tests yielded nothing regarding the pain but did find the enlarged heart. She had multiple painful trigger points in the thoracic and cervical spine. I used the manual spinal nerve block that immediately cut the pain to 3/10. After using a PNT Technique she instantly said that she can breath much easier. Is the patient perfect?

No. But she is significantly better after 3 minutes on the table that she eagerly pays her bill and wants to know when she is to come back. Each visit we have performed fewer procedures and the pain in now at 2/10. She's sleeping better and able to relax and take full breathes."
Jay E. Young, DC Easley, SC

"I've been doing Dr. Kaufman's techniques for 3 years. I can honestly say that miracles are commonplace. Every day, all day, I hear "That's amazing!" The Kaufman Techniques will get you consistent results. The more you learn, the better your patients get. And that is why we all got into healthcare. When I signed up for the September 2010 workshop I called Dr. Kaufman to request the respiration treatment, because I was jealous of the patients that I help with asthma/bronchitis/COPD: they were getting great results, but I still had my own respiratory problems. After a severe injury I had a total chest reconstruction surgery 26 years ago, and have had breathing problems ever since. After treatment at the boot camp, I felt air reaching points of my lungs that I haven't felt in 26 year.
[Subsequent report] *Dr Kaufman worked on my chronic respiratory problems at the October 2010 seminar and my breathing improved more than it had since I had chest surgery 27 years prior. Recently with the allergy season in the Northwest my breathing had started to become significantly labored again. Dr. Kaufman used the new Respiratory Sclerotome Procedure™ at the June 2012 class and I could instantly feel a huge improvement in my breathing. I also feel much clearer mentally. For the past 6 months I'd felt like I was in a constant state of low blood sugar. What a relief!"*
Reuben Mickel, DC Vancouver, WA

"An asthma patient who I've been treating for 1 year presented with wheezing and allergic rhinitis. She is on medication. I utilized the respiratory techniques; with each procedure she felt she was able to breathe better and after the treatment I auscultated her and her wheezing was resolved. Another case is a 9 month old boy who was on steroid therapy 2 weeks ago for possible bronchiolitis. His mother also had a history of asthma and presented with wheezing,

post nasal drip and rattling. I applied the same protocol as above on him and his rattling and wheezing significantly improved and his runny nose stopped. A physical therapist was having acute sinus pain and asthma exacerbation, and I tried meridian bending on her- in seconds she had immediate symptom relief and was pain free. The asthma medication she was taking was not even close."
Jawad Bhatti, MD Midlothian, VA

"I saw a 13 y/o kid that was hit hard in the back with a football. He was taken to the ER and put on an inhaler- he developed a lot of trouble breathing, and was diagnosed with Exercise Induced Asthma. I treated him 3-4 times with the Respiratory Sclerotome Technique™ and his problem completely resolved! He's back running and playing normally."
Terry Williams, DC Ft. Lupton, CO

"Asthma and emphysema have responded remarkably with all of these techniques- The Sclerotome Techniques in one case of severe emphysema/asthma reduced her oxygen usage from 2 1/2 liters per day to 1 liter after the first treatment, and she steadily improved. I've seen perhaps 4 other cases since then with significant stable results. Chronic and severe sinus problems respond quite dramatically, and here in NZ we have a lot of very chronic bronchitis (caused by "other questionable procedures") which is frequently just turned off by the diaphragm reflex and related procedures. I can't thank you enough for all your help with all these people - and for giving me the additional essential means to care for myself and my family as well."
Mark Sinclair, DC Auckland, New Zealand

"A 62 year old woman came to my office with a severe form of asthma, resistant to all medication. Her face was bluish and she had a short, shallow breath. I observed that her shoulders moved very little and when I touch them they were very painful. She couldn't raise her hands for the past 2 years. I treated her shoulders with a simple PNT technique and she immediately began to breathe freely. Her face turned pink in 2 minutes and she could raise her hands over the head. She didn't believe that it was possi-

ble so quickly, but, to tell the truth, neither did I. When I saw her one month later, she was still pain and asthma free."
Dacian Hulber, MD Bucharest, Romania

Thoracic outlet syndrome

"For over 30 years I had been unable to adduct my shoulder more than 90°. In a treatment of less than a minute Dr. Kaufman restored full range of motion, to 160°. That was 5 years ago and I still have full range of my shoulder! Also I recently treated a patient with thoracic outlet syndrome for 25 years that showed remarkable improvement in a few visits."
Kerry Randa, DC Loveland, CO

"I treated a patient with Thoracic Outlet Syndrome of 10 years; in that time, she had flown all over the US and spent almost $100,000 in medical care! She was in severe pain and unable to sleep. After treating her twice with the PNT techniques, she is out of pain and sleeping soundly. She reported that she had been among the worst 25% of Thoracic Outlet Syndrome cases her specialist had seen."
Fred Eckfeld, DC Santa Barbara, CA

"The thoracic outlet case was one of the hardest to treat but she had 50% improvement with 2 treatments. Her neck had minimal ROM but improved to 70° with the cervical protocol."
Jawad Bhatti, MD Midlothian, VA

Post-thoracotomy pain –
Residual pain after surgery

"In 2003-2004 I had multiple surgeries on my lungs, mainly resulting in severe allodynia in my right lower quadrant, loss of motor function in some abdominal structures and hypersensitivity in almost my entire pectoral area. This took me a year to 80% recover from. By becoming a neuromuscular therapist I have luckily been able to 'fix' ALMOST all of the residual pains over the years up to about 95%. Yet, after the first surgery my stamina never returned and I always felt strained due to small aches and pains while per-

forming physical activity. At the October class in 2013 we did PNT on my diaphragm and intercostal muscles and were able to eliminate some trigger points on the spot. The next morning at 5.30 am I decided to go for a run at high altitude here in Denver. After 30 minutes of running I suddenly realized something significant: I was NOT gasping for air, I have had NO twinging in my rib cage whatsoever and I actually felt 'FREE' while exercising for the first time in years!"
Tim van Orsouw, Triggerpoint Therapie. Amsterdam, Netherlands

"The patient had triple bypass surgery in 2003, leaving him with a vertical cheloid scar that went down his entire sternum. He and his wife traveled 150 miles seeking help for intractable pain in the sternum and anterior rib areas. Neither of them could touch his chest without him gasping and withdrawing in pain. Using PNT procedures, I was able to rub the sternum while both of them stared in disbelief. He will be returning to our office for help with other problems, and they've already started making a list of friends and family members they want to send."
Stuart Marmorstein, DC Houston, Texas

"Another patient with breast cancer following a mastectomy had severe pain at the site of the scar. Today her pain and ROM were zero, back to normal since the first treatment."
Jawad Bhatti, MD Midlothian, VA

"A 70 y/o male presenting with chest oppression, shortness of breath and weakness. All these symptoms started after open heart surgery a few years ago. I applied the diaphragm reflex and the sclerotome techniques for about 5 sessions. He gained complete recovery from the afore mentioned symptoms, allowing him to return to his previous job and walk freely without any breathing difficultly, just as he did prior to the heart surgery."
Ran Kalif, LAc. Tel Aviv, Israel

Chapter 13

Abdomen

Acute and chronic abdominal pain

"I have been using Dr. Kaufman's techniques for 5+ years. I see amazing results every day. Three weeks ago I had a 19 year old female come in who was 16 weeks pregnant. She had 10/10 pain from the low back down both legs with intermittent numbness and loss of bowel and bladder function. She was catheterized for 3 days and had not had a bowel movement in 7 days. My first impression was Cauda Equina syndrome, so I sent her and her father to the E.R. They did an M.R.I. to rule out herniated disc and they returned for treatment. I neutralized many trigger points in her abdomen and pelvis/gluteals and legs. After 4 treatments her pain was completely resolved. She was having bowel movements, her catheter was removed and she was able to urinate normally. I have found over and over that when you release pain you allow the body to stop its physiologic response to pain, and that's when the real miracles happen. Thanks again, Dr. Kaufman for changing my life and the lives of my patients."
Reuben Mickel, DC Vancouver, WA

"I've had ICV (abdominal right lower quadrant) pain and tenderness for ~ 13 years, once so severe I went to the Emergency Room thinking it was appendicitis. Dr. Kaufman eliminated that tenderness in seconds with the Pain Control Patterns."
Bobbi Blair-Thompson, DC Huntington Beach, CA

"A 58 y/o male suffering from excruciating LLQ abdominal pain that led him to the emergency room many times. After several colonoscopies and some more tests he was diagnosed as a diverticulitis case and was referred to a GI surgeon. When he first showed up at my clinic he could barely walk straight as the pain was too

strong to bear. After less than 15 minutes, using your manual spinal nerve block procedures, he has regained complete relief. I have treated him several more times, though his pains never returned after the first session. Later on he called to report that his GI specialist said he is not a candidate for surgery anymore."
Ran Kalif, LAc. Tel Aviv, Israel

"My first patient this morning had sharp abdominal cramping after eating pineapple several hours prior. I did the T12 Sclerotome Technique™ and she stated that within 1 minute she felt "unbelievably" better. It's going to be a fun day in the office today. I'm like a kid with a new toy. I used the Sclerotome Technique™ this morning on a patient living with horrible ulcerative colitis for the past 5 years. She is on her last med they will prescribe before they remove her colon. After the sclerotome technique today she said it was the best it has felt in years."
Reuben Mickel, DC Vancouver, WA

"I wanted to tell how much I'm enjoying the latest DVD set on the Adrenal Protocols. I'm continually amazed by how such subtle techniques can produce such dramatic results for my patients. They look at me like I'm from another planet when their abdominal pain disappears after applying a vagus correction to their neck!"
Marcus Smith, M.S., AP. Coral Springs, FL

"It happened again! The day after the 2012 Pain Elimination Class, I experienced the "Kaufman Effect." I now call it "Miracles Monday." Like the patient bent over in acute pain from menstrual cramps experiencing 95% relief in 2 minutes from the new Sclerotome Technique™ ("I love you, Dr. T"). And the patient with Irritable Bowel Syndrome exclaiming, "That's amazing!" as I released abdomen trigger points with the Abdomen Pain Protocol. By now, I shouldn't be surprised because the results are so predictable. Yet it never gets old! Talk about a great ROI!"
Steve Tashiro, M.S., DC Lakewood, CO

"I had two separate women who came to the office, each with a long standing history of frequent episodes of abdominal pain due

to adhesions. One also has scleroderma, and she had just spent 6 hours in the ER after traveling 800 miles from home. The other had pain almost daily, with no effective treatment. Both had tender areas on exam and both had complete resolution of pain with manual spinal nerve blocks. I treated them twice more to be sure but neither had any pain after the first treatment. Needless to say, they were very happy patients!"
Terry Chappell, MD Blufton, OH

GERD (reflux-heartburn)

"A patient with Crohn's disease had severe GERD (heartburn) symptoms with bubbles of possible stomach contents coming up her throat, and severe discomfort in her chest. She had instant relief with the diaphragm reflex. She came in crying and left smiling. (She's also on chemo for Crohns which has not helped for the last 5 months.) "
Jawad Bhatti, MD Midlothian, VA

"I went to the Denver Boot Camp in October 2012. I was a little skeptical about all the testimonies, but decided that if Dr. Kaufman's technique did half of what he claimed, it would be worth the money. After this weekend, I can honestly say this is the best money I have ever spent on a seminar. I was treated for acid reflux at the seminar by Dr. Kaufman, and the next morning was the first morning in 2 years that I did not wake up with reflux. Wow! I would highly recommend this seminar to anyone who cares about helping their patients get well. Follow up 10 days later: I still don't have reflux."
Robert Jeffries, DC Cambridge, OH

Irritable bowel syndrome - chronic constipation - chronic diarrhea - gastroparesis – indigestion

"2 years ago I wrote you a testimonial about a woman with five years of DAILY diarrhea; she's still cured over two years after the first PNT treatments on her abdomen. I never had to touch her

abdomen again. I had such success with that procedure. The only time it didn't work was when the patient ended up being diagnosed with H. Pylori. The effect of PNT on abdominal techniques is almost miraculous. My success rate is around 90%. After using it now for over three years on about 100 "abdominal patients" I felt confident to start advertising to find even more people who need my help. One 16 year old had indigestion after she ate ANYTHING. After about 6-10 sessions she could eat EVERYTHING with no indigestion. Assuming she lives to be 86 that is 70 years of suffering, and needless consumption of side-effect causing medication, that PNT alleviated."
John Clark, DC Newcastle, Ontario, Canada

"The patients are truly amazed that I can change their pain and increase their range of motion in minutes or seconds. Here's just a sample of the success stories: The most amazing success has been with the abdominal techniques. A long-term 70 year-old patient of mine confided in me that she has had a 5-year history of DAILY diarrhea. Nothing helped. After 6 treatments she is back to normal. Another female patient, aged 56, told me she had a long history of heartburn, bloating and diarrhea for 36 years. She could only eat a few bites of food before she felt full. She is back to normal. A 62 year-old woman has had right lower quadrant pain since she was a teenager. After using the ileocecal valve technique only 3 times she is now pain free for the first time in over 40 years. Honestly, you could build a practice around that one technique."
John Clark, DC Newcastle, Ontario, Canada

"Countless cases of digestive disorders improved after a few treatments. I see several patients with abdominal pain daily; this is something that is consistently, remarkably improved. Fatigue and energy deficits are improved with the abdominal procedures. Of course, low back pain and chronic sciatica dramatically improved."
Mark Sinclair, DC Auckland, New Zealand

Residual or recurrent pain after abdominal surgery: cholecystectomy, hernia, c-section, others

"I had chronic right lower quadrant pain with heaviness in the cecum, and pain in the gall bladder area, after a cholecystectomy 7 years ago. It went down my right flank with pain at L5-S1. All symptoms were eliminated after a treatment at the boot camp!"
Clarke Odden, DC Ogden, UT

"One patient had post-surgical abdominal pain for a year, which was totally eliminated in one treatment with the PNT Sclerotome Technique."
Kerry Randa, DC Loveland, CO

*"I've had tightness and tenderness in the abdomen for about 10 years due to surgery. Referral pain was also a problem. Dr. Kaufman treated me and by lunchtime I had **NO tenderness and no referral pain**. He also treated my low-back/sacrum and the pain was gone. I was able to sit through the seminar without pain. I've used Dr. Kaufman's techniques on my clients and have had amazing results. One client has been going to a pain clinic for 10 years and is on 4 different pain medications. After several treatments using PNT her pain is 70% gone and she is off one of her pain meds."*
Sherry Goodrich, LMT. Douglas, WY

"A 30 y/o man presented with multiple abdominal surgeries following acute intestinal blocks due to diverticular formations. When he came he presented these same acute pains previously leading him to the surgeon's operating room. I applied the manual spinal nerve block and the sclerotome techniques. When he came to see me two days later, he reported that soon after he left my clinic the first time, the pains subsided to the point he can hardly fill it. He was so happy to say that its the first time he can recall not ending with another abdominal surgery."
Ran Kalif, LAc. Tel Aviv, Israel

"13 years ago I had 2 major surgeries in a 3 month period. First was for endometriosis (8 ½ hour operation due to complications) followed by a reversal operation for a colostomy (8 ½ hours—

again, complications). This resulted in chronic pain whenever my abdomen was touched. Dr. Kaufman performed the PNT Manual Spinal Nerve Block on an abdominal trigger point. Immediately, there was no more pain. The after-effect was a bit overwhelming since I had been living with this pain for 13 years! Thank you, thank you, thank you!"
Kate Juliano, LMT. Media, PA

"Post-surgical pain in a variety of surgeries has been turned off through your techniques. After our conversation, I immediately used one of the sympathetic techniques for many cases of abdominal pain and problems. It's been very effective."
Mark Sinclair, DC Auckland, New Zealand

"Dr. Kaufman relieved my post-surgical left inguinal hernia pain. I've had a nagging constant chronic pain for 5 years. It took him no time at all to resolve it. 6 month follow up: the pain is still essentially gone."
Patrick Whitaker, DC Belvidere, FL

"I had a patient enter with a pain from an inguinal hernia. He's been in bed for two weeks with excruciating pain on walking. He hobbled in the office and within 20 seconds his palpatory pain was gone! Using PNT techniques he was up and walking without any pain for the first time in weeks. He even noted that the bulge from the hernia had reduced by at least 80%. I really need one of those "Wow, that's Amazing" signs in my office. Since using your techniques I hear that several times daily. I even catch myself saying it!"
Kevin Hay, DC Woodstock, GA

"Dr. Kaufman relieved my post-surgical pain in right lower quadrant. I had hernia surgery in December of 2001 and since then a nagging pain. It took him about 15-30 seconds to absolutely eradicate it."
Bohdan A. Lebedowicz, MD Internal Medicine. Mt Vernon, IL

Chronic pelvic pain – menstrual symptoms

"I had a female patient with severe left inguinal pain. She has a history of difficult and painful endometriosis and gluten intolerance. She told me that it is customary for her to have this type of pain monthly with her cycle. The pain is 7-8 out of ten on a routine basis when this condition flares. I examine her, have her place her finger on the most painful inguinal spot, and I used a PNT procedure. The pain quickly went away. She lights up, in shock, as she is digging into the painful inguinal spot with fingers from both hands trying to find the painful spot she just had and calls over her friend who just started as a new patient, and expressed to her friend that the pain is gone. As the patient is leaving the office I can hear her on the cell phone talking to her husband and joyfully telling him what has happened. Ten minutes later, the husband is calling the office to make an appointment for himself. I'll take those kinds of results every day."
Jay E. Young, DC Easley, SC

"Mood changes, menopausal symptoms, menstrual problems of different types have been significantly eliminated. Every day I see extremity injuries dramatically improved, and colds healed very quickly thru the procedures."
Mark Sinclair, DC Auckland, New Zealand

Urologic problems - kidney stones - chronic interstitial cystitis - testicular pain – pain after vasectomy

"For the past 6 months I've had problems with chronic pain and frequent urination. I've been taking antibiotics every 6-8 weeks due to reoccurrence of these symptoms. After treatment by Dr. Kaufman my condition has improved significantly."
Alan Weber, DC Moody, AL

"A kidney stone had been stuck just below my kidney for 2 months, causing 4 separate visits to the ER and a great deal of agony over many weeks. The surgeon was about to schedule me for surgery. After seeing Dr. Kaufman just one time (and treated with a PNT Manual Spinal Nerve Block Treatment) I was extremely surprised

and delighted the next day when my urologist's X-rays showed that the stone had migrated all the way to the neck of the bladder and was about to leave my system. The stone passed out completely 3 days later. There had been no further pain or bleeding after that one treatment."
Dr. Thomas R. Giles, Ph.D. Denver, CO

"I had a patient with chronic testicular pain for 27 years on a high dose of narcotics. After PNT Meridian Bending his pain decreased to almost zero from an average of 8-9. He was very happy and surprised before he left. A patient with chronic interstitial cystitis had 3 treatments from me so far and for the first time in 10 years her pain dropped to 0 after the 3rd treatment of a Manual Spinal Nerve Block™ and Visceral Impact Procedure™. She's very excited as her average pain scores have dropped so far and her functional life has improved a lot. Please note that she has tried acupuncture before with zero help."
Jawad Bhatti, MD Midlothian, VA

Chapter 14

Back

Acute and chronic back pain –scoliosis

"I did a follow up on a patient with low back pain who was disabled for 2 years with an average pain score of 9-10 <u>with</u> pain meds. On exam her case was more consistent with facet pain and possible radiculopathy. With one treatment of PNT and the low back techniques her score dropped to 2, on average. At her one month follow up today I did a cervical manual spinal nerve block™ and her pain dropped to zero. She's going to go back to work and got a work release from me. I also made her neck 20 years younger with the PNT cervical dynamic lift, which helped her headache to go away completely."
Jawad Bhatti, MD Midlothian, VA

"Dr. Kaufman treated and eliminated trigger points throughout my lumbar-sacral region that had been present for several years and were contributing to left thigh and leg discomfort. As a stand-alone treatment or in addition to your present procedures Dr. Kaufman's techniques are extremely effective. The cervical procedures alone are worth many times over the cost of the DVDs or seminar."
Gord McDiarmid, DC Thamesville, Ontario, Canada

"I had upper back pain for more than 10 years. After one treatment: it was 50% better on the first day. The second day: my pain is gone!"
Lee Huang, LAc. Seattle, WA

"PNT was done on a 35 year old female, who in the last 3 months had chiropractic care, P.T., and a lumbar MRI evaluated by a neurosurgeon. A pain management center did 3 lumbar spinal injections, which increased her pain. After 2 weeks of PNT especially to her piriformis, the patient is now working full time, after 3 months of disability. Another 55 year old female had a lumbar fusion 5

years ago and had received lumbar spinal injections twice a year. PNT was more effective and lasted longer."
Elliot J. Rampulla, MD Diplomat, American Board of Anesthesiology, American Academy of Pain Management, Former Assistant Professor of Anesthesiology and Pain Management at University of South Alabama College of Medicine

"I have had right flank pain for 21-25 years. One of the participants worked on me, doing a psoas lift, and the pain was totally gone in a couple of minutes. I have been having hip pain for 4 weeks—there were several painful points that Dr. Kaufman eliminated in a few seconds. The hip feels better now when walking!"
Kerry Randa, DC Loveland, CO

*"A 70 y/o man had numerous osteoporotic fractures, and was in severe pain for over a year. After I treated him with PNT he stood up, standing straighter and straighter than he had in a year. He said "what the hell?" His pain was GONE for the first time in a year. His wife went back home and referred me ***7*** new patients so far. They live 2 hours away in Stevens Point WI. This is the first time in 50 years of practice that a patient has sent me 7 patients in less than a month. I **was** gonna retire..."*
Charles Raether, DC New Holstein, WI

"My patient had acute low back pain, radiating to both legs. When I saw him at home he was unable to move without severe pain. Utilizing the basic Spinal PNT on two consecutive days he was completely relieved of pain. He was amazed."
Emanuel Stein, MD, cardiologist. Norfolk, VA - Academy of Anti Aging Medicine

*"I got 100% relief of a knife-like stabbing pain in my mid-back, in a treatment that took less than a minute, at the June 2008 Boot Camp. **One year follow up: the pain never returned!** PNT is the most consistent pain relief technique I've ever seen. It really is amazing that something so easy to apply can have such profound results relieving pain and restoring function in patient after patient."*
Reuben Mikel, DC Vancouver, WA

"I've used PNT for about a year now and truly this is an amazing technique light years ahead of its time. One patient was described as being on death's door with chronic low back pain and bedridden for years. After only a few sessions his chronic pain disappeared and he was back to activities of daily living. Friends and family have commented that he's cheated death."
Joey Alcantara, DC Calgary, Alberta, Canada

"I had constant low back pain and stiffness for a year. One treatment (at the bootcamp) and the pain and stiffness was reduced by 90%! Truly amazing!"
Alan Wolchansky, DC St Louis, MO

"Dr. Kaufman's techniques are amazing! I had chronic lumbar pain for 15 years, due to L5 disc thinning and erosion. I needed constant and frequent adjustments. After treatment, my pain has gone and my flexibility is greatly improved! Also for the past 10 years I had chronic pain and limited rotation in the cervical area, and numbness in my right arm. At the seminar, Dr. Kaufman restored 95% cervical rotation and eliminated the numbness in my arm."
Sorina Durante, CMT, CLT. Lakewood, NJ

"I attended the High Speed Practice Growth Seminar October 2011 and Dr. Kaufman treated my upper back pain, which I had had for approximately 15 years. I had been to many other chiropractors with minimal relief. Dr. Kaufman treated me for 2 minutes. I did not feel relief right away. However, a couple of days later when I got home I didn't notice the pain anymore and haven't had it since, 10 months later.
Suhill Samji, DC Vancouver, British Columbia, Canada

"I saw a male 54 years of age with middle back pain and lower back pain. Moderate to severe sharp pain of an unknown mode of onset. His medical doctor tested blood, urine, x-rays and diagnosed arthritis. He began treatments with pain medication without help, then switched to anti-depressants without long lasting help. This patient has been traveling 2 hours to a large city for treatment from a specialist but without long lasting relief. I evalu-

ated the patient and started treatment with the PNT proce-dures. The patient was shocked when we were able to reduce his pain in half with one very simple painless procedure. Each time the patient has had a follow up procedure the results have im-proved, each procedure building on the one before and the pain has been continually improving. He started with 8/10 pain and was seen today for the 9th visit and is now pain free. He is very excited but not as excited as me. He has his life back and I'm tick-led I could play a part in that. It's amazing to be pain free in 3 weeks. "I had a patient in pain that even an implanted spinal stim-ulator didn't help. With PNT I was able to substantially reduce her pain!"
Jay E. Young, DC Easley, SC

"I am a senior athlete.   Back pain has been an off and on chal-lenge for 15 years. Dr. Marvin Wilson, MD relieved my back pain using Dr. Kaufman's techniques last year. I was so impressed that I attended this workshop. Dr. Kaufman relieved more pain in a different area in a matter of seconds. You have to experience this to believe it!"
Kathleen Hunter Levy, LCSW. Topeka, KS

"I saw a female with mid back pain; she saw a chiropractor for 6 months with what he thought was a "rib out". She had no con-sistent relief. After 6 sessions of various PNT techniques- the PAIN IS GONE AND STAYED GONE!!!
Derick Russell, PT. Chicago, IL

"Two months ago I experienced an episode of debilitating low back pain that required spending 3 days in bed, and a few weeks of limited mobility. Flying to Dr. Kaufman's seminar was very un-comfortable and aggravated the pain and stiffness in my back. By the 2nd day of the seminar, after Dr. Kaufman and some classmates worked on some trigger points, my low back felt more comfortable than it's felt in years."
Jim Stegenga, LAc. Olympia, WA

"I had a T12 compression fracture 9 months ago and have had nagging left sided low back pain since. After PNT treatment my pain was quickly reduced by 50%. I am 70% better today (2nd day) of the seminar after the Sclerotome Treatment by Dr. Kaufman."
Dr. Atul K. Shah, MD, Radiologist. Mumbai, India

"I had a 260 lb, 6"2" race car driver patient today who has not slept well in a month due to severe low back pain with radiation down his leg. It was my office mate's patient. He's been in about eight big crashes, so where do I start. First, I just did a quick disc move which is both diagnostic and the treatment. Nothing. Then, I just went right to PNT on the piriformis, SI joints and psoas. His points shut off quickly. Before I did any kind of AK work-up, he was walking around like nothing happened."
Aleae Pennette, DC Santa Rosa, CA

"I came to the June 2012 seminar with chronic right-sided cervical to lower thoracic tightness and trigger points. Also, I had a moving vehicle accident the week before the seminar. After 2 minutes of PNT I felt a 'lightening' of the upper trapezius muscles, less of a desire to 'self-adjust' and I was told I was immediately sitting up more erect and held my head higher. One hour later I found it much easier to maintain proper posture."
Mark Milleville, PT. Wheatfield, NY

"The patients are truly amazed that I can change their pain and increase their range of motion in minutes or seconds. Here's just a sample of the success stories: My absolute favorite patient came in yesterday. She is 93 years-old and has been suffering with spinal pain for 'many years.' She also has right trapezius and right gluteal pain. The MDs have written her off as having 'degenerative osteoarthritis' and told her to 'live with it.' She's 80-90% better. She's saying that she's 'thrilled.' It's very rewarding to be able to help people like that. It's such a great feeling to walk into a room with a patient knowing that there's a huge likelihood they're going to use the term, 'wow, that's amazing.'" Every DC, PT, MD, and acupuncturist should have these tools in their toolbox. For massage therapists, PNT could be the ENTIRE toolbox."
John Clark, DC Newcastle, Ontario, Canada

"One of my long time patients came in not being able to sleep for the past three nights due to pain in their upper back. The patient was taking a medication for their advanced leukemia and the pain was due to the muscles reacting to the process. Thankfully I was able to reduce the muscle pain using Dr. Kaufman's PNT Facet Syndrome/ Spinal Fixation 2 way Reflexes enough to where they could breathe deeply with no pain and get up and lie down on the table with no pain. The second visit two days later they reported they were able to sleep through the night (and the edema in their legs reduced temporarily). They were very grateful for this as they go through their difficult process. I cannot express my gratitude for being able to help someone in so much pain."
Robert Jeffrey, DC, LAc. Los Angeles, CA

Sciatica - bulging disks – herniated disks – nerve compression

"I had a 42 year old female yesterday come in with left side sciatic pain with radiation of pain into the left thigh and buttock. Used the spinal nerve blocks and meridian bending with gall bladder reflex points and she noted a 90% improvement following my 6 minute treatment."
Dean Odmark, DC San Antonio, TX

"3 weeks ago a patient asked me if I could help his 87 year-old grandfather who was suffering from sciatica. He'd been to his MD and meds didn't help. His x-rays revealed DDD and DJD. After one treatment, yes one, he reported 50% reduction in pain. After several visits he was totally asymptomatic! Thanks for making me look good!"
Jim Monk, DC Chickasha, OK

"An MRI shows herniation on my L3 to L5 discs. I have had low back pain--right sciatica for the past 2 years intermittently. Dr. Kaufman treated me at the seminar, and I felt instant relief."
Robert L. Fish, DC Jackson, MI

"I'm seeing an 86 year old male with sciatica. He had been getting regular injections of lidocaine into trigger points for the pain. The relief would last two days. Our first visit removed pain for that amount of time with no injection. The second lasted even longer. He is happy to come in once or twice a week if necessary instead of being injected."
Aleae Pennette, DC Santa Rosa, CA

"I saw a 12 year old boy who was diagnosed with lumbar plexopathy 2 -3 years ago. This boy had only one session of PNT when I neutralized his psoas trigger point with the agonist technique. At that time I was in the initial phases of learning PNT My nurse called his home today and his dad is reporting 90% relief at one month, after just the one PNT application. His hip hiking is completely resolved. Please note he had an EMG at University of Jackson confirming the lumbar plexopathy diagnosis.
[He] …is now off baclofen. He still has some back pain and tight hamstrings. I did the PNT Meridian Bending; he had significant improvement in his gait and started walking pain free. His flexion was 20° bilaterally at the hip with knee in extension before the treatment and became 90° degrees after the procedure."
Jawad Bhatti, MD Midlothian, VA

"I have been getting FANTASTIC RESULTS!!! This stuff is so effective it's the only treatment I usually use for pain. A patient with lateral femoral cutaneous nerve pain was almost all better after treatment. A patient with severe knee arthritis had dramatic improvement-the pain hasn't returned 7 mos. later. Some patients call me "the magician" or "magic fingers"
Derick Russell, PT. Oak Park, IL

"After attending the June class, I returned and treated a patient who had residual big toe weakness and numbness in his leg due to a 10 year-old lumbar disc injury. He had been treated by me and other chiropractors in the past with adjustments but with the addition of PNT, he and I were both thrilled to discover that he had recovered strength in his big toe and normal sensation in most of his leg, for the first time. I also treated a woman at a sporting event who complained of back pain that she had had for <u>40</u> years.

The next morning she arrived to tell me that her 40-year-old back pain was completely gone!"
Rachel Richards, DC San Diego, CA

"I saw a 40 year old female with disc protrusion on MRI, left side radiculopathy and a palpable painful floating knot just left of the L2 spinous process. Her pain was 6/10. With PNT the pain was reduced in half. Her left SI joint was producing the most pain. I did a manual spinal nerve block and immediately her pain went to zero. When she got off the table she was a flat zero out of ten."
Jay E. Young, DC Easley, SC

"I had a patient come in from New York with sciatica. She had been to 5 different practitioners, and no one had been able to help her. Using PNT, after about 15 minutes it was gone. She also had tinnitus for over 40 years and had 90% relief on the one treatment, I only got to see her the one time."
Aaron Flickstein, DC Edina, MN

Sacroiliac joint and coccyx (tail bone) pain

"Dr. Kaufman treated my right posterior sacral/iliac joint problem. Something I had been fighting, unsuccessfully, for over a decade. In a matter of minutes, the pain was <u>GONE</u>!! I am very excited for a future without lower back pain."
Terry Billings, DDS. Metairie, LA

"I've had left sided sacral segment pain off and mostly on for years, that was virtually eliminated after a brief PNT treatment. Dr. Kaufman also quickly relieved my left hip pain of 55 years with a treatment that took a few minutes."
Timothy Binder, DC, N.D., LAc. Hamilton, MT

"The Sclerotome Techniques make it very easy to handle pelvic, SI joint and sacral pain. I've also had great results with a number of patients with limited shoulder abduction using the Paradoxical Muscle Reflex™. Awesome!"
Stuart Marmorstein, DC Houston, TX

"At the June 2012 PNT seminar, Dr. Kaufman addressed my right sacroiliac joint which has had chronic tenderness and reduced range of movement for 10-15 years. After performing 2-3 simple procedures, I noted the tenderness was greatly reduced. Later, I tested the range of motion while stretching. The improvement was unmistakable. I could perform much fuller stretch with much less pain in the sacroiliac."
Mark Seitz, DC Dayton, OH

*"I had a L/SI joint/piriformis/Iliotibial band pain for about 3 months, possibly due to a fall on stairs. Dr. Kaufman worked on all 3 areas and I am **wildly better!** I cannot believe that no one is teaching us this technique in medical school. My relief was instantaneous. I have had OMT, prolotherapy, trigger point injections and have done yoga--all to no avail and this treatment worked in 5 seconds. It's crazy. I must learn the mechanism and technique."*
Dorothy Pedtke, D.O. Grand Rapids, MI

"A 65 y/o male with post trauma tail bone pains, leaving him unable to sit and lay down in most positions. He went to several pain clinics but gained no relief. I saw him only twice, applying PNT on sacral trigger points and using the Gracilis Reflex Technique. He recovered completely and was actually able to sit after the first session."
Ran Kalif, LAc. Tel Aviv, Israel

Chapter 15
Upper extremities

Frozen shoulder

"A 50 y/o woman with an 18 month frozen shoulder with less than 30 degrees abduction ROM, no internal or external rotation ROM and less than 40 degrees extension ROM. She came with her husband with a thick medical documents file, after seeing numerous shoulder specialists and attending several rehab clinics. I learned from them that this issue has completely turned their life upside down. It will sound pretentious but it's the absolute truth to say, that after applying the joint repositioning on her, she has regained full ROM both abducting and extending her shoulder, while regaining almost 50% in lateral and internal rotation- and that is after less than 10 minutes when she first entered the treatment room. She looked at her husband and they both started to cry, hugging each other. My assistants, some are with me more than 15 years, couldn't believe their eyes. And so did I..., she came for a few more short sessions after which she returned to a normal life routine. An 85 y/o male with 50 years frozen shoulder (his shoulder problem equals my age...) treated with the PNT Cervical Protocol and joint repositioning. He has regained full range of motion in less than a month (he shows up only once a week). His daughter sent him to me though he didn't believe it's even possible to gain relief after half a century of suffering. To tell you the truth, at first, neither did I."
Ran Kalif, LAc. Tel Aviv, Israel

"I treated my 79 year old mom's frozen shoulder. Her condition was a result of a mastectomy performed 26 years ago. It was so bad at times that she had to hold a spoon with her left hand; the right didn't flex to get the spoon to the level of her mouth. In three treatments her right shoulder flexion is now 160 degrees, and has stayed this way for a month.
Galina Semyonova, LAc. New York, NY

"Dr. Dan Michalec worked on my frozen shoulder with PNT and it is much better. I have suffered with it for 9 months and the pain had been almost unbearable."
Gloria Perkins (Wife of Elbert Perkins, DC) New Braunfels, TX

Other chronic shoulder pain – residual pain after shoulder surgery

"I had a pain raising my left arm (shoulder alducha) just before the end of the <u>ROM</u> the pain was significant but not debilitating. Just one procedure completely obliterated the problem (eliminated the pain). Thank you very much."
Michael Konig, DC   New York, NY

"I injured my right shoulder in chiropractic school. It has been a nagging injury since. Dr. Kaufman worked on my shoulder /trap yesterday and today it is 90% better. I went home and worked on my husband's left knee. He has had patellar tendonitis from teaching/playing tennis and after about 5-10 minutes of working on his knee using the Agonist method he was able to walk upstairs without pain! Thank you for teaching this work!"
Carrie Stone, DC   Lincoln, NE

"I have had moderate restriction and mild pain in my right shoulder for over twenty years since shoulder surgery, despite previous attempts to correct the condition (Chiropractic, physiotherapy, etc). In just one treatment by Dr. Kaufman of approximately one minute duration, to my own and everyone's amazement, full range of motion was restored to my shoulder. This was after twenty years! This is truly medical magic! Thank you Dr. Kaufman!"
Jeffery Marston, DC Mandeville, LA

"I had pain in motion while twisting and laterally raising my arm. Dr. Kaufman treated me for 2 minutes and I could raise my arm without any pain through full range of motion during the application of one of his techniques. I have had this problem for about 1.5 years."
Ivan Petrarnichki, Personal Trainer. Varna, Bulgaria

"I had fantastic results with a left shoulder problem. At the October 2009 Bootcamp I couldn't raise my arm more than 90°. After the first and only treatment, I could raise it 160 ° and now in June, 2010, **my arm is 180° with just a slight pain toward the end of abduction**. *Also, I find my vision is better after neutralizing trigger areas in my neck. My experience with your approach has been phenomenal. I'm now especially sure and confident when taking care of people! "*
André Laplante, DC Gatineau, Québec, Canada

"My shoulder pain of 3 years significantly improved after only a few minutes of work. I was legitimately surprised at the speed of improvement even though I've been doing PNT for a while now! The manual spinal nerve blocks have completely changed my treatment approach, almost overnight. It is downright scary how fast this stuff works on a good portion of patients. This was easily the best purchase I've ever made in the realm of technique DVDS."
Nick Dimovski, DC Chicago, IL

"I had an exacerbation of scapula and shoulder pain that I've had on and off for 10 years. During that time, I'd tried massage, ART and chiropractic care with limited success. I was treated during the seminar and had the sensation of increased blood flow into the arm. After the treatment, the pain was gone and there was no more grinding!"
Rachel Richards, DC San Diego, CA

"I've suffered chronic neck and shoulder pain for 15 years, from various sports and car accident injuries. I usually have to get aggressive chiropractic adjustments in order to get relief. After just 2 minutes of treatment, I feel great!"
Tom Grant, DC Salt Lake City, UT

"I've had trapezius pain for 2 years that radiated into my shoulders, bilaterally. I had complete and quick relief after the treatment. It really is amazing!"
Vicki Lumpkin, DC Lubbock, TX

"I've suffered pain in the right shoulder for 2 years, pain that radiated down to my arm. The treatment restored my range of motion without any pain. 2 days before the seminar, I injured my lower back during my morning exercise routine. I could not bend forward or sit. After treatment I am 100% pain free!"
Helen Law, LAc. Princeton, NJ

"For over 30 years I had been unable to adduct my shoulder more than 90°. In a treatment of less than a minute Dr. Kaufman restored full range of motion, to 160°. That was 5 years ago, and as you can see, I still have full range of my shoulder! Also I recently treated a patient with thoracic outlet syndrome for 25 years that showed remarkable improvement in a few visits."
Kerry Randa, DC Loveland, CO

"An extremely intelligent and fit woman has been unable to play tennis for months, due to a shoulder problem. She had done all the usual things that included orthopedic surgeons and traditional physical therapy. After 3 visits that were highlighted by the Sclerotome Technique, she is back on the court. My biggest problem with the Sclerotome Technique™ is, it neutralizes trigger points so quickly and often, that I often wonder if the patients are making this stuff up."
Steven Lavitan, DC, LAc. former columnist, Dynamic Chiropractic. Paramus, NJ

"At the June class, Dr. Kaufman treated my left shoulder pain of approximately 9 months duration. The pain was worse on abduction to 90 degrees; on external rotation there was a very sharp pain. It was also worse when lifting my 22 month old son and doing weight training. The treatment with Joint Re-positioning Techniques, and reducing trigger points in the left infraspinatus using the Sclerotome Techniques reduced the pain dramatically."
Suhill Samji, DC Vancouver, British Columbia, Canada

"My patient had pain in the arm and shoulder for more than 20 years and was unable to lift her arm up to her head. Her range of movement was about 60%. In less than a minute, after doing the

Kaufman Upper Extremity Protocol, she was able to raise arm completely up."
Valerie O'Rourke, R.N. Elk Grove, CA

"I had a longstanding injury to the right shoulder that caused shoulder and elbow pain to occur on abducting my shoulder beyond 120 degrees. Within 2 minutes of applying one of Dr. Kaufman's techniques in the classroom, I could raise the arm beyond straight up (180 degrees) with no shoulder or elbow pain. Dr. Kaufman treated me at the seminar for low back pain, which abated with the utmost speed. Not bad, after 3 chiropractors in my city could only give me temporary relief, at best."
Stuart Marmorstein, DC Houston, TX

"My chronic left upper trapezius pain was gone in a matter of seconds. I have had this pain for 25 years after a rugby injury in college and have been treated with chiropractic, massage, acupuncture, etc and none of those brought the degree of relief that Dr. Kaufman gave in a matter of seconds."
Sean Felton, DC   Kansas City, MO

"I had a Work comp shoulder patient who works 13 hrs. per day with shoulder pain and restriction; 2 sessions of your shoulder techniques and her ROM is normal, and pain is very little."
Derick Russell, PT. Chicago, IL

"I had severe deltoid pain and limitation of motion in my shoulder for 6-8 months. I regained full range of motion without pain after treatment!"
Herbert Dees, DC Farmington, NM

"For 3 months I couldn't sleep on my right side due to shoulder pain. I also had pain on raising the arm. A boot camp attendee did the Pain Elimination Grid technique and the pain disappeared! I'm also using the techniques with great success."
Marvin Wilson, MD, Vascular Surgeon. Topeka, KS

"I was treated in the seminar for my left shoulder pain and neck pain. My shoulder has had pain on abduction for 6 months. Dr.

Kaufman did a few techniques, and my shoulder pain on abduction was gone, and my neck range of movement was also increased in a few minutes."
Margaret Mei, MD New York, NY

"I had pain in my right acromio-clavicular joint for two months. Dr. Kaufman used the Pain Grid technique on two spots. The trigger points cleared immediately and the shoulder was the best it had been in two months within a few minutes, even though I had been treated by a chiropractor and three other body workers back home."
Stuart Marmorstein, DC Houston, TX

"I used the advanced meridian bending for shoulder ROM on a patient with moderate to severe osteoarthritis, who had a complete range of motion increase from 90 to 180°. One patient with severe osteoarthritis of the shoulder (who already had one shoulder replacement done) had 90% pain relief. I've had lots of other success stories similar to these cases."
Jawad Bhatti, MD Midlothian, VA

"I could not extend my left arm more than 30° without extreme shooting pain. I've had this since a fall 3 months prior to class. Dr. Kaufman treated me in class, using the shoulder protocol. In a short time I was able to raise my arm over my head with no pain. The next day I still had no pain. I was able to raise my arm over my head, no limitation."
Peggy Gray, LMT. Colorado Springs, CO

"I had a patient with many operations on his left shoulder. He had a claw hand on his left side, and he's left handed. He had severe pain through his neck, down his arm and into his fingers, and also scapular and rib pain. He also had a massive amount of scar tissue from the surgeries. I did the Sympathetic Protocols on his Inferior Mesenteric Ganglion and Stellate Ganglion reflexes and the pain in his neck and down into his fingers disappeared. I then did the Mandibular Reflex and there was a dramatic improvement in the scapular and rib pain."
David Walsh, MD   Mobile, AL

Rotator cuff injuries

"The patient had severe left shoulder pain although he had steroid injections just last week. He had rotator cuff surgery previous to that. His PROM [passive range of motion] *was 60 degrees in passive abduction. After 2 minutes of treatment he reported no pain, and displayed full range of motion both passive and active. He said I was a "Voodoo Doctor" which in my younger (more sensitive) years would have been insulting, but I took it as a compliment. He brought his wife in, today, who suffers from ankylosing spondylitis. She was very skeptical. But not after her first treatment!"*
Rick L. Townsend, DC, NMD, LAc. St. Robert, MO

"I have had right shoulder pain due to a rotator cuff injury for approximately 20 years. PNT techniques in the last 2 years have improved both the pain and range of motion significantly. Today, however, I experienced the best range of motion ever secondary to a subscapularis technique! Even my small residual shoulder pain has disappeared."
Bonnie Friehling, MD Columbia, MO

"A patient with a severe rotator cuff tear with only 5 ° of movement was improved to 90° abduction on the first session with PNT At a 1 week follow up she still had 70° of abduction, up from 5°but decreased from 90° after her first treatment. PNT gave her another 40 degrees of pain free abduction today. When I asked her if she wants any pain meds she said no. Please note she has not been able to do anything with this arm for the last six months. Another patient, age 39, with MVA [motor vehicle accident] *who's been seeing me for 5 months with history of a rotator cuff tear and severe back pain. She'd received trigger point and botox injections in the past with minimal relief and is on Lyrica, Vicodin and Flexeril therapy. I applied PNT for her back and a manual spinal nerve block™ for her shoulder with 90% relief. It seems like she was very happy."*
Jawad Bhatti, MD Midlothian, VA

"I had rotator cuff surgery on my left shoulder. I had torn the subscapularis muscle away from the proximal humerus and the surgeon reattached with 2 helix screws and cord. They also repaired the subscapularis labrum and repaired the medial bicepital tendon. After PT, I was unable to reach behind my back or raise my arm in abduction past shoulder height. I had a severe trigger point in my left pectoral muscle that was eliminated using the PNT Brain Reflex Techniques™. After one treatment by Dr. Kaufman, I was able to have full ROM in my left shoulder both in horizontal abduction and internal rotation. Thank you Dr. Kaufman for your dedication to the healing profession."
Alan J. Weber, DC   Moody, AL

Epicondilitis –
Tennis/golfer elbow

"While attending the June 2012 Pain Elimination Seminar I was treated by Dr. Theo Peters, MD, for right lateral epicondylitis. Prior to the treatment I had sharp pain for the past four weeks in my elbow and was unable to straighten my arm. After one treatment my pain has significantly reduced and I have pain free motion in my elbow."
Alan J. Weber, DC Moody, AL

"A patient with bilateral severe epicondylitis got 90% relief."
Jawad Bhatti, MD Midlothian, VA

"Since the June Boot Camp, I have been using the techniques on every patient at my office the very next day. To see the reaction of the patients as the tender points disappear is priceless. One example is a patient with a chronic epicondylitis on the right side. He had an extremely tender point in his forearm extensors just below the elbow. I did a Pain Control Pattern and it went to zero pain. You could see the confused and shocked look on his face as it happened. As he was leaving he said his elbow was feeling better already from the treatment. It took only about 2 minutes! I am impressed! It was a great and extremely useful seminar. Next time I will book the flight out the next day to take advantage of

your staying so late on the last day to make sure everyone got it. I know that is exhausting and appreciate your commitment to helping us."
Robert Jeffrey, DC Los Angeles, CA

"On Thursday I worked on a woman's elbows with PNT When I saw her last night I planned on doing it again. Well, before I started working she said that she was pretty impressed with the results and I asked her why. She said after the one treatment she was able to rub her eye...she had not been able to TOUCH her eye for 14 years!(for some reason she hadn't mentioned that before) Needless to say we are both very excited!"
Connie Danner, N.D. Amarillo, TX

Wrist pain – Carpal tunnel syndrome – Hand/finger pain

"A follow up of 3 cases of carpal tunnel syndrome showed 2 of them treated with PNT reported 100% overall pain relief with one treatment at one month. The other patient is a physician with documented mild right and mild to moderate left CTS [carpal tunnel syndrome]. *The right side got 90 % relief with only mild relief on the left, 3 weeks after treatment."*
Jawad Bhatti, MD Midlothian, VA

*"In just 3 hours, I learned enough to relieve the pain right away from a 4 year-old injury to my husband's right wrist. I went back to my room at the hotel where the seminar was being held, excited to try the new techniques on him. He wasn't even able to brush his hair without wrist pain. He had **NO** pain when we finished!"*
Michele Chambers, LMT. 29 Palms, CA

"A 58 year old male injured his wrist working on his car. Three months after that, he still had pain and swelling. He was given cortisone shot in his wrist. He had no relief from pain with the shot. Finally, 6 months after his injury, his wife brought him in to see me. Using your techniques, after the first visit he said his wrist was 75% better. And then he said, "That's amazing". As he

left the waiting room, he stopped and told my next patient about his 'miracle'."
Eleanor Devinney, DC Denver, CO

"Dr. Kaufman treated my right thumb pain....75% improvement in a matter of 2 minutes!! Thumb pain is not good for a dentist. An MD wanted to do surgery. Now surgery is not needed and I feel great!"
Terry Billings, DDS. Metairie, LA

"With all the classes I've attended with Dr. Kaufman, I still learn incredibly useful new information in each class. The respiratory protocol has been very successful in helping people breathe. I've had right hip pain and knee pain nearly a year, limited, painful range of motion. Dr. Kaufman eliminated several trigger points in a very short time and the knee pain is gone, immediately. I've had a burning nerve pain in the right thumb on elbow and thumb extension. Dr. Kaufman eliminated the burning with a treatment that took less than one minute."
Kerry Randa, DC   Loveland, CO

"Thanks for a great Boot Camp last week-end. I've worked with the material all week. I was the one who was constantly saying "Amazing!" It was incredible. Necks, low back, legs, heels, fingers. Wow! I really had a lot more fun in the office this week. A 71 year old male fell and severely injured his little finger. He tore the tendon. A surgical repair was suggested. When he came in for treatment, he could not bend his finger at all. Using PNT protocols, he could bend his finger 75% right away. After a few treatments he had 100% use of his little finger. He decided not to do the surgical repair."
Eleanor Devinney, DC Denver, CO

*"I'd given my notice of retirement to the clinic where I work. After many years of health issues, multiple surgeries, then a rear end accident that severely injured my right hand/ thumb I was resigned to retiring and going on Disability. I was depressed, emotionally crushed. At the June 2011 seminar, Dr. Kaufman treated me with the **Mandibular Reflex Technique**. I was amazed at the immediate*

release of pain in the upper traps and my rib cage. What blew me away though was the fact that as I went to go sit down, I realized that the horrendous pain I had in my thumbs (which I had told Dr. K nothing about) was gone. Totally gone. For over 1 ½ years I had continuously dealt with this pain. It caused me to limit bodywork to one session a day, to get sometimes daily chiropractic adjustments, and use the laser therapy at the office several times a week. The only medical option given to me was to give up bodywork. The pain stayed away completely for 4 days. It was significantly diminished when it returned somewhat, and as time went on it again eased to the point that I'd have to remind myself that I'd ever been injured. I withdrew my retirement notice, went back to work, and increased my bodywork hours. The PNT techniques are amazing. I've found that at least 95% of my clientele benefit from PNT"
Peggy Gray, LMT. Colorado Springs, CO

Chapter 16
Lower extremities

Hip pain - ankilosing spondilitis

"The patient had severe left shoulder pain although he had steroid injections just last week. He had rotator cuff surgery previous to that. His PROM was 60 degrees in passive abduction. After 2 minutes of treatment he reported no pain, and displayed full range of motion both passive and active. He said I was a "Voodoo Doctor" which in my younger (more sensitive) years would have been insulting, but I took it as a compliment. He brought his wife in, today, who suffers from ankylosing spondylitis. She was very skeptical. But not after her first treatment!"
Rick L. Townsend, DC, NMD, LAc. St. Robert, MO

*"After watching the first 3 Manual Spinal Nerve Block DVDs, I had a 50 year old with hip dysplasia who had been in **severe pain for 2 years** report 75% pain reduction in 3 treatments. An 80 year old with severe trochanter pain GONE in 30 seconds. A 75 year old with **severe low back pain reports 80% relief in 2 minutes**. I've seen **many upper trapezius trigger points gone in less than 1 minute,** too many to count. One patient told me "to go do that Voodoo that you do so well." This after 4 upper back trigger points disappeared in about 1 minute."*
Jim Monk, DC Chickasha, OK

*"I've had pain for over 20 years at the C7-T1 level that resolved in a very short time after treatment at the June Boot Camp. I also had bilateral hip pain for months that I thought was from DJD [degenerative joint disease], but x-ray did not show any degenerative changes. I was having trouble walking. After treatment the pain was gone on the spot; I have no more hip pain. **One year follow up: both problems never returned after that treatment!"***
Terry Williams, DC Ft Lupton, CO

"The cost of all the DVDs I've bought from you has already been far far outweighed by the value my clients and myself have received. How much is it worth that last night my patient walked into my office without her cane????!!!! Up and down the steps too. We have been working to avoid hip surgery for a year and she has this week given up her dependence on her cane!!!   WOW!! I knew it was coming but I wasn't quite sure she knew. How much is that worth to me, but truly how much is that value to her?? I don't think we can put a price on it. That's all from the PNT techniques!!
Connie Danner, N.D. Amarillo, TX

"I have been playing with the info from your Sclerotome DVDs with some excellent results so far. I had a new patient come in today with severe hip pain who interestingly could not flex her knee, even 5 degrees. I figured this was a real test for the paradoxical muscle reflex. I applied it to the quads and nothing happened. Then I applied it to the psoas and instantaneously she was able to bring her heel to her buttocks. We were both speechless!!! That was the highlight of my day and I am sure hers as well. Thanks, Stephen!!! "She had 6 months of no flexion at all in the knee, all the time. She was getting locked up intermittently for the last 5 years, getting more and more frequent. Her hip is still an issue but greatly improved with PNT! Went from 8-10 on visual analog scale for hip pain on walking to averaging (1-3) on ambulation."
Daniel J Bank, DC Queensland, Australia

"One patient who fell from a horse 10 years ago was on high dose of methadone and Klonipen therapy with severe limitation of hip flexion to 20°. PNT dropped her pain down to zero; with tears in her eyes she told me she's never felt pain free before, even with methadone. Her pain score never dropped below 7. Her positive limited SLR before the treatment went to 90° of flexion.
I just had a patient with ruptured quadriceps tendon barely able to walk with severe pain above the knee. He had a visible deformity above the knee of the quadriceps tendon and ROM was limited on flexion, secondary to severe pain. Advanced meridian bending with

knee flexion gave him 90% relief and he left my clinic on his feet walking pain free."
Jawad Bhatti, MD Midlothian, VA

"A 90 year old healthy, active female fell in a parking lot putting groceries in her car. She landed on her left gluteal area. She could not get up on her own. She went to the ER, was x-rayed, no frac-tures were found. A week later, she came into my office. She was hunched over her walker and shuffling her feet in small steps. She had a knot in her gluteal area the size of a fist. After using Dr. Kaufman's PNT Techniques, she was able to stand up and walk with small steps without shuffling. She said her pain was reduced by at least 50%. I then attended Dr. Kaufman's 2012 Boot Camp where he introduced the new Sclerotome Techniques, before I saw her again. She walked into the office without her walker, not up-right, with an altered gait, and on pain meds at night. I used the new Sclerotome Techniques™ with her. When she left the office, she was upright, and had no pain, and her gait was much im-proved. She said, "This is unbelievable! I feel so much better. At my age, I didn't think I could recover from this fall. The Sclero-tome Techniques are easy to use and very effective. I love this new work!"
Eleanor DeVinny, DC Denver, CO

Groin and leg pain – osteoarthritis – degenerative joint disease –iliotibial band syndrome

"Dr. Kaufman worked on my right leg and relieved several trigger points which have been present for 2-3 years (I had been having pain, weakness and muscle spasm). My leg feels normal on sitting and standing (now)."
Brian Briggs, MD Minot, ND

"I had a lady come in today with groin pain on lifting the left leg. She had no palpable trigger points and the only remarkable find-ing was a weak psoas on the side of the groin pain. Instead of strengthening the psoas I tried a pinwheel test on the legs for sen-sation and there was no sensation over the L4 dermatome on the right side. I applied the manual spinal nerve block to L4 on the

right side for 20 seconds. Immediately she had full sensation of the right dermatome and a strengthened left psoas along with no groin pain!"
Daniel J. Bank, DC Queensland, Australia

"The week before I came to the class, I had worked out and done a lot of challenging leg work. My calves were super tight and sensitive during the seminar. A girl I don't even know (someone new to the technique) used the Sclerotome Technique™ to work on the involved muscles. Immediately there was improvement, and the next morning I am tight but the pain has gone from a 9 to a 2. Myself, my husband and our 10 children and our 5 (so far) grandchildren are pain free. Come on, what is that valued at????"
Connie Danner, N.D. Amarillo, TX

"62 y/o female with right leg pain for 3 years. Is giving notice at work because she cannot perform the duties. Had knee surgery to release the peroneal nerve. The surgeon described the surgery as "textbook". Pain persists, patient now has to use cane. Goes to pain clinic where she is fit with a spine stimulator. Still has to use cane with doubtful reduction in pain. Comes for acupuncture in desperation (her husband is a retired ortho Surgeon). I prescribe PNT First treatment: 70% reduction in pain and patient leaves office carrying the cane!"
Rick L. Townsend, DC, NMD, LAc. St. Robert, MO

"I injured my left medial knee after a fall and had acute pain in the medial femoral condyle when walking and this had been four weeks. Prior to this I had been running 4-5 miles, 5 days per week and was then unable to run. Dr Kaufman treated me at the seminar on Saturday, using the Grid Technique. After the treatment I honestly thought he had missed something because there was still very little change in my condition. Upon waking up on Sunday morning, the pain had reduced by approximately 65% and walking was easier. The take home point on this is that sometimes we have to be patient and give the body a chance to heal."
Alan J. Weber, DC Moody, AL

Tight hamstrings

"After learning the techniques in class, a first time doc was able to increase my ROM in hamstrings and abductors by about 30%. Previously there was pain upon motion. After treatment, there was none. My energy increased and I experienced more clarity for learning."
Aleae Pennette, DC Santa Rosa, CA

"Dr. Kaufman successfully performed a quick procedure to 'dramatically increase hamstring length' on my right hamstrings which have been tight for as long as I can remember. Ever since I learned about trigger points, I had been able to TEMPORARILY relieve this tightness using trigger point massage and dry needling, but those results never survived the night. After waking up Monday morning after the class, for some strange reason the first thing I did upon waking was to test my hamstring length by performing a fingertip-to-toe stretch. To my surprise I could grasp my right foot with my knee straight, without having to 'warm-up' first. Working with PNT has really become a game-changer in way I now address pain and trigger points, period. I will be looking forward to be part of this new movement in natural healing."
Tim van Orsouw, Triggerpoint Therapie. Amsterdam, Netherlands.

Knee pain

"Today, Dr. Kaufman addressed some chronic pain in my right knee which I have had for 10 years. The initial trauma disrupted the MCL [medial collateral ligament] *and medial meniscus. Ever since then, I've had sporadically occurring right medial knee pain. It has recently flared up again. Dr. Kaufman found and neutralized 3 pain points in the area. Within two hours I have noted the recent symptom set has decreased substantially when standing and walking. Based on previous experiences with Dr. Kaufman, I know to expect a long term, fundamental improvement in my knee."*
Mark Seitz, DC Dayton, OH

"I just had a patient in that I have been treating for right medial knee pain. She is all better from using mostly the grid technique and meridian bending. I asked her today, "By the way, how long have you had that pain?" "Since I was 14". She is 61 years old. Yup, 47 years of pain, GONE!"
John Clark, DC Newcastle, Ontario, Canada

"I injured my right shoulder in chiropractic school. It has been a nagging injury since. Dr. Kaufman worked on my shoulder/trap yesterday and today it is 90% better. I went home and worked on my husband's left knee. He has had patellar tendonitis from teaching/playing tennis and after about 5-10 minutes of working on his knee using the Agonist method he was able to walk upstairs without pain! Thank you for teaching this work!"
Carrie Stone, DC Lincoln, NE

"I have been getting FANTASTIC RESULTS!!! This stuff is so effective it's the only treatment I usually use for pain. A patient with lateral femoral cutaneous nerve pain was almost all better after treatment. A patient with severe knee arthritis had dramatic improvement-the pain hasn't returned 7 mos. later. Some patients call me "the magician" or "magic fingers"
Derick Russell, PT. Oak Park, IL

"The Pain Neutralization Techniques are incredible, this is so much fun to see the look on people's faces when you shut down a major pain. Almost too many cases to list. I had a patient last week with knee pain for a year, and couldn't walk well. I did the PNT and there was absolutely no pain. Walking is now painless! It was amazing!"
Kerry Randa, DC Loveland, CO

"In October of 2004, I injured my left lateral meniscus. The subsequent MRI revealed a mild tear. You treated the knee for pain at the fibular head and surrounding area and the pain went from VERY TENDER on palpation to at least 95% improved. Flexion increased immediately by 20-30 degrees. The restriction and tightness was all gone!"
Marvin R. Terry, DC Orlando, FL

"What was most impressive to me was my self-treatment on my own lateral knee pain. After a simple procedure, the pain is gone. Also, your treatment of a Doc with significant shoulder dysfunction blew me away. Very impressive!"
Michael Moralez, DC Delavan, WI

"I saw a patient who had both knees replaced, with severe pain in the knees and lower back pain. I treated all the trigger points above and below the knee joint- the difference was night and day."
Jay E. Young, DC   Easley, SC

"I also wanted to share a personal testimony about my daughter. She is 23 and recently torn the meniscus in her right knee. After weeks on crutches and taking pain medication she decided to give mom a try to see if I could help her (unfortunately my children have more confidence in western medicine at this time in their lives but they are slowly coming around to the holistic side). After only one treatment her pain was reduced by 80% and held until the next treatment. After the second treatment her pain was completely gone. She was totally amazed! Your techniques are truly AMAZING!! I use your techniques on just about everyone that comes through the door and my success rate in alleviating pain has dramatically increased. I look forward to continuing to learn and apply more of your techniques, as so many people can benefit from them."
Stephanie Ward, AP. Homestead, FL

"Yesterday Dr. Kaufman performed the equivalent of a "total knee replacement" on my right knee: 20 years ago I tore the right medial meniscus. I had surgery and a portion of the meniscus was cut out. 2 weeks ago, I reinjured it. I turned and there was a loud pop in my right knee. I couldn't bear weight on it, and it swelled up. After Dr. Kaufman graciously worked on me in class, I have no pain in my right knee—it's gone! So after class I worked my left knee in a similar fashion and that pain is gone. This stuff is wild and amazing!"
P. J. Zaramskas, LAc. Pollock Pines, CA

"Since November 2011 (7 months) I have had left knee pain that did not allow me to squat past 20% range. (I had a surgery scheduled in 4 days that I cancelled to await a stem cell procedure to regrow the cartilage.) An MRI showed I had a full thickness chondral defect. Dr. Kaufman treated the trigger points surrounding the knee. One hour after the treatment I was very anxious to test a single leg squat. On my own, I attempted it and to my complete amazement I was able to perform a full single leg squat without pain! I don't remember being able to do this even prior to me hurting my knee. I will no longer be looking into any surgical intervention and am planning to call my orthopedist to try and lighten his surgical load. Wow, that's amazing!!"
Mark Milleville, PT. Wheatfield, NY

"One 82 year old female patient had knee pain and a burning sensation into her feet. Her secondary complaint was indigestion and constipation (for as long as she can remember). All these symptoms are dramatically improved (90%). The knee pain was recreated by pressing on trigger points on the medial knees in an area where you normally don't expect to find muscle trigger points (but as you said at the seminar a better definition of a trigger point is where it is tender, regardless of whether or not there is a muscle belly in that location - that was one of the pearls of the seminar). What's really cool about this patient is that she has already had both her knees replaced! So from a medical perspective, everything that could be done, had already been done. But, her continuing pain was from the surrounding soft tissue, obviously not from the knee joints. I had another patient in last week- she's very overweight, with osteoarthritis of the right knee confirmed by x-ray. Her MD told her to take Celebrex and wait for a knee replacement. She could not stand for longer than a couple of minutes due to knee pain. This has been the case for years. After one session of PNT (meridian bending) she was remarkably improved, and amazed. A couple more sessions likely will cure her too."
John Clark, DC Newcastle, Ontario, Canada

"Follow up on one of the patients with severe lateral knee pain and who was on crutches had an overall 80% relief with one treatment of PNT She's now walking without crutches and has can-

celled her surgery. I just had a patient who left crying with happiness. She gave me an euphoric rush. She had severe knee pain for ten years. This was her second treatment and her pain was zero today for the first time in ten years. She has x ray proven moderate to severe osteoarthritis of the knees. I felt my endorphins releasing from this and I guess we all hope for these moments. I asked myself, "why do people use recreational drugs .....they don't need them! You get much higher from seeing people so happy!

I had a patient with knee pain from severe osteoarthritis with leg bowing. Using the Manual Spinal Nerve Blocks™ I was able to bring his pain down to zero. This amazed me.

A patient with a hip prosthesis and knee pain had about 50% improvement with 3 treatments using combinations of joint gliding and PNT"

Jawad Bhatti, MD Midlothian, VA

"The patients are truly amazed that I can change their pain and increase their range of motion in minutes or seconds. Here's just a sample of the success stories.

A 17 year-old young man with a 5 year history of bilateral knee pain is now pain free. A 50 year-old woman who had persistent pain for over 2 years after knee surgery is now pain free."

John Clark, DC   Newcastle, Ontario, Canada

"Every day I see several patients with knee injuries. Whether with or without surgery- I don't remember any that have not responded significantly in both reduction of pain and increased of range of motion from the PNT techniques."

Mark Sinclair, DC Auckland, New Zealand

Osgood-Schlatter's disease

"My son suffered Osgood-Schlatter's Disease causing chronic bilateral knee pain for over a year. He couldn't run, jump, or play football without using compression bandages. He was living by icing and Advil after every game, but not anymore. After one treatment using PNT and manual spinal nerve blocks by Dr. Kaufman, he no longer has any pain. If I hadn't heard him com-

plain every day for over a year, I wouldn't have believed he ever had it. Truly, it's a miracle."
Debbie Lantz, R.N., Nursing Manager, Rheumatology and Neurology, Kaiser Permanente. Denver, CO

Ankle pain – Achilles tendinitis

"I had patient referred from a podiatrist with ankle pain and with plantar flexion due to "arthritis in the ankle- bone on bone". After 2 sessions of using the grid techniques, the pain is gone and stayed gone!"
Derick Russell, PT. Chicago, IL

I twisted my right ankle 2 weeks ago stepping out of my car, and went down to the ground in pain. There was swelling around the lateral ankle. I had deep pain. Dr. Kaufman did PNT on my ankle. My ankle was pain free at once. About 3 hours later I noticed I was able to trot upstairs on tiptoe. And, I am fully able to sit 'Indian-style' with zero difficulty and zero pain. I have full range of motion."
Jessie Conley, RN. Mount Vernon, WA

"I had a female patient with severe Achilles tendonitis. Her MD told her she had reduced blood flow. She uses a cane and heavy duty ankle brace, with an antalgic gait pattern. I treated her 6-7 times with PNT techniques- her pain is gone, she now uses no cane, no ankle brace, and has a normalized gait!!!"
Derick Russell, PT. Chicago, IL

Plantar fasciitis

"I also had a debilitating and fairly acute plantar fasciitis in my left foot. I had only had it for a week, but it was interfering with my ability to walk, and sometimes hurt when there was no pressure on the foot. His work drastically reduced the severity of the pain, and after taking some supplements to help inflammation and icing it, the pain was gone within two days. I rode my bicycle for half an hour this morning."
Stuart Marmorstein, DC Houston, TX

"I had Plantar Fascitis pain for 4 months. Dr. Kaufman treated me using the Grid Technique. The pain reduced to almost imperceptible. Kudos for PNT"
Dale Ruemping, DDS. Seattle, WA

*"Treating the neck muscles reduced pain and increased ROM in over 20 patients. Metatarsalgia and severe plantar fasciitis was relieved in 3 patients instantly. These patients were in **severe** pain. 2 patients with chronic pain on morphine daily reported 80% improvement in pain."*
Jawad Bhatti, MD Midlothian, VA

'Many, many cases of plantar fascitis (heel or toe or wherever) have been corrected in 1-4 treatments."
Mark Sinclair, DC Auckland, New Zealand

Foot pain

"I had a work comp patient with foot pain from a fractured metatarsal; she walked with a limp. After 2 treatments of PNT, her pain is gone, he gait is normal, and she's returned back to regular duty!!!!"
Derick Russell, PT. Chicago, IL

The patients are truly amazed that I can change their pain and increase their range of motion in minutes or seconds. Here's just a sample of the success stories.
A 47 year-old woman with 20 years of pain following a fractured foot is now pain free after only a few treatments.
John Clark, DC Newcastle, Ontario, Canada

Residual or recurrent pain
after lower extremity surgery

"I saw a 75-year-old female patient from South Texas (Rio Grande Valley) yesterday. She complained of pain in the knee (where she'd had surgery years back) and numbness in the calf and

foot. Using the new sciatica sclerotome work and the PNT two-way facet reflexes along with other PNT procedures, all of the pain and numbness was gone after the treatment. I saw her for other issues today and she told me that she hadn't needed to take any medication for pain and could easily walk to the kitchen."
Stuart Marmorstein, DC   Houston, TX

"I had constant neuropathic pain radiating from my hip and pelvis to my groin and front of my leg due to surgical complications 4 years ago. To my amazement, the constant shooting pain eased, then stopped after treatment at the seminar. This pain has limited my lifestyle for the past four years, and I'd tried everything traditional and alternative medicine had to offer with limited results. This is most wonderful for someone who had been told either I could learn how to live with it (as I'd done) or become a nonstop user of painkillers! More than one treatment may be needed, but what an AMAZING result for just a few moments of effort. 'Wow!'"
Christy Wilson, LMT. Dallas, TX

"One patient had foot pain secondary to ankle fracture following an open reduction, internal fixation surgery a week ago. Her pain came down to 2 from 10 with manual spinal nerve blocks. The hydrocodone she was taking could only bring it down to 7."
Jawad Bhatti, MD Midlothian, VA

"A 60 y/o male underwent a medial meniscus surgery, following which he remained disabled to the point he could not fully flex and extend his knee. Walking without a stick wasn't even an option. After many months of unsuccessful rehabs and seeing many knee ortho specialists, he came to see me without any expectations. Now, after less than 3 months, he has returned to play tennis and even won 2 national senior contests, not to mention that he doesn't use a stick anymore and walks about completely normally."
Ran Kalif, LAc. Tel Aviv, Israel

"One of my best cases was a 13 year old, who came to me about 2 ½ years after a large picture fell on him and the glass severed his Achilles. He had surgery to repair it when he was 10, and since

that point, had experienced pain everyday, all the time. He is an athlete, and if he got hit in that area while playing football, he was on the ground. He would not even let his mom touch the area. The first time he laid on the table and I applied very light pressure to the area, he flinched. I examined his calf, which had some tender spots, and just using the agonist technique, was able to treat those. The next morning his mom texted me and said her son was so excited, because for the first time, he got out of bed and put his foot on the floor, and didn't have pain. As a mom, she is thinking in her head that her son has 60, 70, 80 years of pain. She was beside herself excited. He came back and it took 2 maybe 3 treatments, for all of the tender areas to stay gone. We have watched his Achilles decrease in swelling and narrow down, to where it now matches his other Achilles."
Carrie Carter, PT.   Little Rock, AR

Phantom limb pain

"I had a patient with diabetes and phantom limb pain of 10 (on a scale of 1-10) secondary to below the knee amputation. The pain level dropped to zero after the PNT application. On a follow up, the patient reports zero phantom pain since the first treatment.
I just had a 29 year old patient with a left below the knee amputation on Lortab therapy with severe hip pain and sciatica for years on the residual limb, and phantom limb pain on the left. He had a prosthesis which was few inches short. He got 100% percent relief on the sciatica 60% relief for phantom pain."
Jawad Bhatti, MD Midlothian, VA

Chapter 17
Reported functional disorders

Hypertension

"I've been getting amazing results for HTN. I've had numerous patients have very significant drops of blood pressure with one of the advanced PNT techniques. 13 out of 16 patients with hypertension had a substantial drop in blood pressure; the average BP in 11 patients dropped from 158/89 to 131/75!

One patient with hypertensive urgency had a drop of 70 points systolic on the spot! A follow up on this patient was that she did not have to go to the ER as her blood pressure numbers stayed low. Usually with symptomatic HTN urgency cases I admit them to hospital for 24 hours but in her case it was not needed.

I had another patient with BP 172/90 who dropped to 120/80 - please remember he has been on BP medication for 4 years and never been that low.

One lady with anxiety levels of 10 dropped to 0. She told me "doc, it felt like I just took a tranquilizer".
Jawad Bhatti, MD Midlothian, VA

"I've seen quite a few cases of normalized blood pressure, eliminating the need for medication. Really, many different conditions respond."
Mark Sinclair, DC Auckland, New Zealand

Adrenal fatigue – low energy

"A 56-year-old female patient presented with symptoms of hypoglycemia, a condition that she has contended with for years. She reported that she couldn't take adrenal nutritional supplements, because they tended to keep her awake at night, leaving her with

even less energy. She felt markedly better after applying just part of the new adrenal protocol."
Stuart Marmorstein, DC Houston, TX

"Dr. Kaufman performed the Adrenal Rejuvenation protocol on me at the seminar on June 9, 2013. I have been suffering with adrenal insufficiency and lack of energy for the past ten years. During the treatment I felt a surge in energy and my circulation and metabolism were given a boost also. I feel a calm energy and look forward to my renewed sense of well-being. Thank you Dr. Kaufman."
Sorina Durante, CMT, CLT, Lakewood, NJ

Rhinitis –sinusitis

"A patient has been seeing me for 4 years with severe allergic rhinitis who takes at least 3-4 rounds of steroids per year. Today I treated her with a rublite on her sinuses with complete relief. She did not ask for any medicine after the treatment and sounded very surprised.
I had a gentleman with acute sinusitis and pink eye requesting medications. I applied your rub lite procedure and the pain level of 10 out of 10 in the sinuses and eye dropped to 0 out of 10. His pink eye also had rapid improvement."
Jawad Bhatti, MD Midlothian, VA

Fibromyalgia

"43 out of 49 low back pain patients had rapid relief! 34 out of 37 neck pain patients got immediate reduction of pain! **2 fibromyalgia patients had full relief**. 5 patients had good relief of abdominal pain. 7 headache patients had full relief."
Jawad Bhatti, MD Midlothian, VA

"A few weeks ago, a fellow flew in to Houston from Mangalore, India for help with fibromyalgia, headaches and related problems. Based on the distance he had traveled, I worked with him on several consecutive days. He had so much relief and felt so normal, he

told me he wished I could travel to Mangalore (population 10 million) to treat people. I told him it would make more sense for him to send someone to America for training so that there would be someone available there all the time. He plans to return to Houston in October for follow up care, but left here with the sense that he could lead a normally active and comfortable life. With my next three weeks booked solid, I don't think I can take the time off from practice here to journey to India.
Stuart Marmorstein, DC Houston, TX

Reflex sympathetic dystrophy

*"I had a patient with **Reflex Sympathetic Dystrophy** and arachnoiditis since 1992. She was down to 97 lbs, in severe pain, and barely functioning. She'd had both knees replaced, the left one twice, bringing on the RSD. Her pain management specialist inserted a neurostimulator in her back surgically to help block the extreme pain. The strongest pain medication didn't help. She couldn't stand for anyone to even lay a hand on her legs. Using PNT, I was able to eliminate almost all of the pain in her legs in a couple of treatments, and the best part is that it held!"*
Don Gay, DC Florence, CO

Neurologic deficits

"I saw an approximately 60 year old female actress: This beautiful actress does a stage act as Marilyn Monroe. Six months ago while hospitalized for a hernia operation she had pneumonia. She had produced a blood clot below her lung that traveled to create a stroke while in the hospital. She saw me three weeks ago on two consecutive days. Her gait improved. Her left hand changed from plastic looking to a normal looking hand. She is excited and looking forward to going back to work on stage again. Triple Wows!"
Fred Eckfeld, DC Santa Barbara, CA

"I treated a bodybuilder whose left arm hand and fingers were paralyzed, since fracturing 4 cervical vertebrae 2 years ago. He'd had surgery at that time and was in hospital for 8 weeks. He

couldn't move his fingers. 40 doctors and neurologists had told him he would never regain use of his arm and hand. He had zero deep tendon reflexes in his triceps and biceps. His fingers, biceps and triceps were absolutely paralyzed.

On the first visit, using meridian bending and other PNT techniques, he regained full strength in his arm muscles, and almost full movement in his fingers. All his deep tendon reflexes came back. Feeling returned to his hand. His hand had looked very pale; almost full color came back after treatment. Both he and his wife started crying; his wife continued to cry for 10 minutes. This patient was referred in by a young girl who'd had severe migraines for 8 years. Her migraines stopped after 2 PNT treatments."

Marcus Seuthe DC Black Forest, Baierbsronn, Germany

Peripheral neuropathy

"*I had a chronic inflammatory demyelinating polyneuropathy (CIDP) patient scheduled today which has progressed to an extent where she was unable to walk. She is very reluctant to take medicines. She has received 2 rounds of IV gamma globulins which gave her motor nerves some improvement. I did PNT meridian bending on her and she told me that it felt weird as it seemed her sensations were coming back and her burning pain had disappeared. She walked in with a cane and left without it. Please note the above diagnosis are confirmed and documented with serial NCS and EMG studies.*"

Jawad Bhatti, MD Midlothian, VA

"*A patient with idiopathic peripheral neuropathy for the last 17 years came to me for acupuncture treatment. She is on methadone to control the pain but even so the pain would be unbearable by the end of a day's work. While acupuncture dramatically improved her numbness, she would still have pain by the end of a day. I used meridian bending to neutralize trigger points in her lower legs and **the pain turned off at once**! We were both shocked and on follow up have found the pain relief to last about 5 days. And the technique is so simple that I showed her son how to do it between office*

visits. She has dropped her narcotic dosage for the first time in 17 years and is planning to drop it again. I can't wait to use the new techniques I learned at the seminar for neuropathy."
Jim Stegenga, LAc. Olympia, WA

"What a fabulous seminar!!! I have never been to a seminar that the presenter just kept giving and giving and giving great information, especially past the usual scheduled time. I really appreciate all your extra time and effort. I have a patient that had severe neuropathy of both feet for several years. It was so severe that he could hardly walk and to touch his feet would cause excruciating pain. The color of his feet was a deep purple and red, with protruding veins in the ankle. After approximately six treatments using your techniques and nutritional supplementations he is now able to not only walk comfortably but the pain is almost completely gone. Needless to say he is beyond happy and I credit it to your very effective techniques."
Stephanie Ward, AP. Homestead, FL

"I saw a 50 year old male patient who had years of left posterior shoulder pain as well as right sided facial numbness. He had many approaches and treatments to no avail. As he came to me for a third treatment in a six day period he exclaimed the shoulder pain was gone and his face felt normal again. Big WOW!!"
Fred Eckfeld, DC Santa Barbara, CA

"Prior to the October Bootcamp, I had symptoms of peripheral neuropathy: burning in my feet, and stiffness in both hands during the middle of the night and upon waking. Medically, we weren't sure if it was residual from myopathy secondary to a statin drug or the beginning of diabetes. Debbie Powell, P.T., treated me in class and the burning in my feet resolved, as well as complete relaxation. The burning did not return that afternoon or the next day which is the first time in a year I have tolerated sitting. Later, she treated Trigger Points throughout the spine and stiffness was not there when I awoke the next day. It is wonderful to find relief to symptoms that I did not think were musculoskeletal problems. However, it is even more wonderful to be relieved of the worry about what was causing the symptoms! This information opens

many opportunities to help our patients that we never dreamed could be so fast!"
Beth Whitehead, PT. Jackson, AL

Sleep disorder

"I treated a patient for sleep apnea and he had significant improvement in his symptoms instantly, with better breathing and he was not snoring as loudly. Please note that he had rhinoplasty done 4-5 years ago. Now the doctors were talking about another surgery as he not able to tolerate CPAP/BIPAP. His wife reports a significant reduction of sleep apnea after the procedures."
Jawad Bhatti, MD Midlothian, VA

Chapter 18
Other organ dysfunctions

"2 miracles today: A patient had crushing knee pain and severe edema eliminated on the spot. The lady was able to walk again, which was not possible for 5 weeks. She was receiving cortisone injections and acupuncture from a local orthopedist who said it was due to "arthrosis" - her pain got worse and worse. I used the Pain Grid and Meridian Bending and that was the end of that. No pain at the end of the session, full range of motion.

The 2nd was even more of a miracle. A 78 year old lady had kidney function of 20% with severe edema in both legs and cardiac insufficiency. I did the Visceral Impact Procedures and she called me tonight very excited. She had to run to the bathroom at least 10 times and lost about 4 Liters through her urinary tract. Medication had stopped working to eliminate her excess fluid. We treated her and the edema was gone for the 1ˢᵗ time in 3 years."

Marcus Seuthe, DC Black Forest, Baierbsronn, Germany

Chapter 19
Acute pain syndromes

"I had a patient with L4-5 paraspinal abscess with severe pain of 10/10. I drained the abscess and applied a manual spinal nerve block™ with 80 % relief. She had about 50 cc of pus which we were able to drain.

I had a patient with pain of 10/10 from a knee abscess. I gave him a manual spinal nerve block™ and his knee pain dropped to zero. Then I performed an incision and drainage on him. He's 27 years old and had back pain and carpal tunnel syndrome which also completely resolved with PNT So these techniques do work when there is pathology secondary to infection.

A patient with a displaced ankle fracture whose first cast failed and had recasting done last week with pain 9 out of a possible 10 dropped down to zero with a manual spinal block. It seems like spinal blocks have very good response for acute pain with pathology."

Jawad Bhatti, MD Midlothian, VA

"I had acute back pain for 3 days with insidious onset. I could barely bend forward. After Dr. K used the Paradoxical Muscle Reflex, there was a great increase in ROM from waist, right away- and reduced back pain – within an hour!"

Robert Good, DC Santa Barbara, CA

Chapter 20
Veterinary medicine

"These techniques are spectacular! As a veterinarian I tried PNT on my 15 year-old dog, "Rex". After a few techniques Rex seemed a different dog. He was able to stand quickly and walked with a new freedom. The next day my wife called me, in tears, and relayed that Rex was running in the back yard, like a 2 year-old dog, galloping full strides. I was thinking his days on earth were numbered. I've used the techniques on numerous clients' animals with similar impressive results.

I used the Sclerotome Technique today on a greyhound - he was limping on the right front leg, C5, 6, 7 discs collapsing; he was crying out with pain on mild cervical palpation. After the procedure I pressed very hard just to satisfy my curiosity; there was absolutely no pain. I re treated a 2nd time just because I pressed the trigger pts again. The dog was 90% sound on day 2; hopefully we got the remaining 10% today. 3 weeks later: the greyhound is still going strong. I treat almost every canine I see using your techniques."
James E. Watson, DVM. Denver, CO

"Five months ago our 11-year-old West Highland Terrier injured his right shoulder. My wife took him to the vet, who could find nothing wrong. Two weeks ago, he re-injured his shoulder and I decided to try a cervical manual spinal nerve block one night before he went to bed. Next morning he was no longer limping (he limped for three days prior)! It was a great feeling to help our dog!"
Edgar F Ruble, DC Schaumburg, IL

Chapter 21
Miscellaneous reports

"On Monday, June 10, 2013 at my office I was excited to try out some of the new things Dr. Kaufman demonstrated over the weekend at his Pain Elimination Protocols Mentor Class. As it turns out one of my long time patients came in that day due to not being able to sleep for the past three nights due to pain in the upper back. The patient was taking a medication for their advanced leukemia and the pain was due to the muscles reacting to the process. Thankfully I was able to reduce the muscle pain using Dr. Kaufman's Facet Syndrome/ Spinal Fixation 2 way Reflexes enough to where they could breathe deeply with no pain and get up and lie down on the table with no pain. The second visit two days later they reported they were able to sleep through the night (and the edema in their legs reduced temporarily). They were very grateful for this as they go through their difficult process. Thank you Steve. I cannot express my gratitude enough for being able to help someone in so much pain."
Robert Jeffrey, DC Los Angeles, CA

"I had one patient with severe bone pain from melanoma- gone, after treatment. Many, many others with severe, chronic pain- gone! Not only were the results on other patients/physicians stunning, but also the treatment I had: in 2-3 seconds, all of my own trigger points and facet pain disappeared! "It's amazing!" and "It's gone!" are exactly what I hear from my own patients: it's a hoot! Your techniques have added a HUGE new dimension to my practice; they put the fun back in, after 43 years."
David Walsh, MD Mobile, AL

"After utilizing the basic PNT protocol on my local pain specialist MD, he has been so impressed with the results he has referred up to 5 patients a day to my practice! He has been to many other pain specialists in other areas of the country and locally with no results. After only a few PNT treatments, he is comfortable at work as well

as other activities. He is now working toward returning to a very strenuous tennis routine.
Brian Osborne, LAc. Plattsburgh, NY

"A 38 y/o woman in her 36th week of pregnancy presented with a fetus in breech position. Her OB/GYN doctor told her she will need a cesarean, because he tried to perform physical flip under US scanning and couldn't make it. I treated her with PNT The next day she called to report that soon after leaving my clinic she felt a movement inside her, so she rushed to the doctor's office to perform a US scanning which showed her fetus now in a normal position. Later on she naturally delivered a healthy baby."
Ran Kalif, LAc. Tel Aviv, Israel

"3 years ago I was having severe cramping in my arms whenever I'd work for 10 minutes; I was going to have to give up practice. I was looking at retiring from being a chiropractor. Dr. Kaufman treated me one time at a seminar, and I haven't had any problems since. This is my 5th PNT seminar, I fly here from the Netherlands." **Adrian Jasperse, DC Netherlands**

*"While I've been using your methods to some degree since meeting you several years ago, my use was really more "superficial" or "haphazard"; I certainly did not achieve real excellence. Recognizing that I was still missing some pieces, (despite good results) I began studying your DVDs and using your procedures on every patient, in preparation for this seminar. This has been a truly inspiring experience. **I simply never realized how great your protocols are.** I'm now able to achieve much better results than ever before-and fast. Patients are often amazed and really love their improvement, and also the gentle way this comes about. I feel a new passion about my practice and my commitment to help as many people as possible. As a long-time AK practitioner (along with other related techniques such as TBM, ART, NET, CRA, BodyTalk), **I love being able to get** away from the more conceptual explanations (which most patients don't get anyway) **to the bottom line of pain-light touch-no pain**. I'm very grateful for your work."*
Frederick Mindel, DC New York, NY

"I was a new patient in this very successful chiropractor's office. My lower back was really out. I had great difficulty putting on my socks, sitting down, standing up or lying down. After a brief treatment I walked out of there, with the pain gone. He said 'that was the Kaufman Technique,' and I said to myself, 'I need to dedicate my life to learning that, because that works!'"
Jessie Conley, RN. Mount Vernon, WA

"The self-treatment techniques alone are worth far more than the price of the seminar!"
Dale Reumping, D.D.S. Tahoma, WA

"The seminar was amazing. The techniques were very easy to learn and implement. I witnessed many miracles as about 60 of the participants were treated by Dr. Kaufman for chronic pain. I started using these procedures on Monday morning at 9:00 a.m. The feedback using Dr. Kaufman's techniques has been amazing from my patients. The term "wow, that's amazing" has actually started to get a little old! My own knee pain of about 2 years duration was gone and stayed gone after I treated myself at the seminar (3 months ago). Dr. K has been sending me letters for 3 years. Quite frankly, they all sounded too good to be true. I didn't believe it possible that trigger points could be turned off in seconds with neurological reflexes. What really convinced me to come to the seminar was all the positive feedback from previous attendees. I figured they must all be telling the truth or he's a gifted writer of fake testimonials. Either way, I wanted to find out. Honestly, of all the professional development I've done in my 16 year career, this was the most useful and practical technique seminar of them all. The patients are truly amazed that I can change their pain and increase their range of motion in minutes or seconds."
John Clark, DC Newcastle, Ontario, Canada

"I have been getting the most amazing results. These techniques are astounding and I have helped many clients who have had chronic pain for years. It's incredible how tight muscles and trigger points just melt under my fingers. People come in that can barely move and leave feeling such relief. I had one client tell me he hasn't had this much pain relief in 15 years. I've been getting

lots of referrals. During the seminar I had pain in my neck and low back. I worked on myself and the pain slowly went away. I also had Dr. Kaufman work on my arm which has been very sore around the medial elbow. The pain went away in seconds."
Gayla Norgren, LMT. Platteville, CO

"My son has had seizures for about 5 years. I treated his back, neck, and head using PNT I noticed that he became more calm, and doesn't have seizures anymore. Knowing that lots of autistic children have seizures, I worked on a couple of them. Their parents noticed significant differences in their behavior- they became so much calmer. Another experience (good one!) I treated a patient with Lyme disease. She slept better and it definitely released chronic pain she had for more than 20 years. I use PNT on my mom, who has hip (bone-to-bone) pain and has tried laser and injections—PNT had the <u>BEST</u> (!!!) results! It is amazing!"
Ingrid Chegai, PT. Santa Cruz, CA

In the average patient I see, what used to take 15 treatments now takes 3-4. With most musculoskeletal problems it takes 3-4 treatments with Dr. Kaufman's techniques to get 80-100% improvement. Patients generally feel 70-100% improvement during the first treatment. It is fun to be a patient hero!"
Galina Semyonova, LAc. New York, NY

"I just wanted to drop you a note to tell you how marvelously pleased I am with the material presented in the sets of DVDs I recently purchased. Colleagues and patients alike are just as impressed with the actual work. On many occasions, I have detected an immediate palpable release at the trigger point at the exact moment the correction is applied. This is WAAAAAAYYYY COOOOLL !!!! This is very exciting to me. It is reframing my entire experience as an acupuncturist. And I've been an acupuncturist for 18 years."
Marcus Smith, M.S., AP. Coral Springs, FL

"Wow! And wow again! As dramatic as the literature for the Manual Spinal Nerve Block™ may seem, if anything it's understated. My experience over the past months with patient after patient

has been phenomenal! Nasty trigger points (like upper trap) and chronic pain patterns literally do disappear in a treatment that takes 15-30 seconds using this breakthrough. I've gained such confidence in my ability to handle really tough pain syndromes I'm calling those intractable patients whom I've exhausted my options with and discharged- I feel now there's hope for them!"
Steve Tashiro, DC Lakewood, CO

"Once Dr. Kaufman started showing the techniques I gasped: 'Oh my God, he could teach 3rd graders to be healers.' The techniques are so astoundingly simple, yet profoundly effective. It's a revolution in healing. I could see its application in class but once I got back to work the reality set in. Before I was starting to feel like a mechanic, cranking and twisting, popping and pulling. Now I feel like a magician, waving a magic wand."
Chris Tusken, DC Loveland, CO

"Thank you, thank you! My wife says PNT is the best technique ever—the first time we can shut down one of her headaches immediately! My regular patients are just as impressed! "Amazing" is now an everyday word in my practice. These new procedures are the most powerful techniques that I've learned in 34 years! You've truly taken it over the top this time! Any technique this simple, yet this powerful, is truly going to go wild."
Don Gay, DC Florence, CO

"Dr Kaufman's techniques are so simple and effective, they'll turn even the most chronic skeptic into a believer. I work in a high volume clinic seeing between 160-190 patients/week and we use the techniques on almost every patient. How effective are they? Well, we're booked 3 weeks out now and have patients begging to be seen. Learn the techniques and start getting the results you've always dreamed about!"
Joseph Giacona, LAc. Brooklyn, NY

"The techniques continue to be phenomenal, even after several years! They've made my treatments so much more effective and patients love the fact it's not painful. My only complaint is my patient volume has gotten out of hand due to referrals and I can't

handle all the people that want to see me. I just got a much bigger office, hired an associate and two secretaries- my practice is exploding out of control!"
Ken Andes, L.Ac, DOM. Suffern, NY

"This is some of the most exciting stuff I've seen in years. Thanks to you, I'm swamped (with patient referrals)! I've never had these kinds of results with anything. PNT is amazing. (Like you promised) I have patients saying "Wow! That's amazing!" all the time. You've made my practice fun & exciting again which is particularly rewarding as this is my 27th year in practice!! I had epicondylitis for 3 months and after a 2 minute treatment my pain and limited ROM is totally gone!! The Pain Control Patterns (PCP) have produced amazing results. I had an 87 y.o. man, who's had back surgery, open heart surgery, DJD, DDD. I told him that he wasn't a candidate for spinal manipulation but we could use the PCP. This man was severely depressed from constant pain made worse by even minimal physical activity. I did the PCP and the grid technique and his pain has gone from a 10 to 1-2! I taught my son the sciatic technique over the phone-in 5 minutes, his girlfriend's severe sciatica was GONE! Several patients have had a large drop in blood pressure with the hypertension protocol."
James Monk, DC Chickasha, OK

"I'm having many "AMAZING" results from PNT, MSNB and the other techniques since last summer's Boot Camp. I've had 3 patients who had shingles and did the MSNB technique with great results. "In 1990, I had the opportunity to train with Janet Travell, MD, as part of my acupuncture training. Since then, I've been using acupuncture trigger point therapy as a major part of my practice. With the techniques I've learned during the Boot Camp, my use of needles for treating trigger points has become minimal."
Peter Goldberg, D.A., LAc Great Barrington, MA

"I can't emphasize enough how important it is that my fellow colleagues take this work. The public at large needs this work desperately. The cervical work is absolutely great. On returning to practice I did an experiment and told patients that I would be doing a different type of work on their necks, a non-manipulative ap-

proach. Out of the hundreds I did this on, only one wanted a standard cervical manipulation. The feedback was great on the new techniques and everyone loved it. <u>It still produces a better result on the cervical spine than any other technique I have used in the last 20 years.</u> The low back techniques are incredible. I have been able to resolve several stubborn cases...."
Dean Odmark, DC San Antonio, Texas

"I watched Dr. Kaufman treat over 50 MDs. at the A.C.A.M. conference. After treatment, each doctor felt at least 80% better; many close to 100% improvement. The next day, I asked 12 of them how they were. 11 of 12 felt much better or amazingly better."
Gerard Pesca, N.D. Phoenix, AZ

"I like the fact that something as profound as this treatment can be done easily with bare hands in our current age of high-cost technology health care."
Kamal Karl, MD Napier, New Zealand

"Every pain you addressed was eliminated in a matter of seconds. Neck pain gone, back pain gone. The shoulder pain and (oh yes!) range of motion of the doctor sitting next to me was almost unbelievable—right before our eyes."
Dard Muhammad, LAc. Houston, TX

"These amazing techniques have been a phenomenal addition to the practice. For anyone 'on the fence' about buying your DVD's, they should ask themselves one question: 'Could I treat patients with one hand and still provide effective pain relief?' Well, I broke my right hand and practiced PNT hours after I got my cast. I practiced this way for three weeks, <u>with no loss of income</u>. Not only should doctors learn these techniques for the amazing pain relief, it was a great insurance policy for what may have been a devastating injury for me."
Tom Kramer, C.A. Red Lion, PA

"Dr. Kaufman held a roomful of MD's and D.O.'s spellbound with his non-invasive techniques to relieve pain instantly. He created a groundswell to invite him back to more and more."
Terry Chappell, MD Blufton, Ohio. Past president, American College for Advancement in Medicine, founder, International College of Integrative Medicine

"The Pain Neutralization Techniques are incredible, it's so much fun to see the look on people's faces as you shut down major pain."
Kerry Randa, DC Loveland, CO

"I am a Doctor of Physical Therapy, and I've been in private practice since 1993 seeing outpatient neuromusculoskeletal disorders. I've trained in most manual therapy systems and a multitude of orthopedic PT methodologies. I'm a constant learner and avid practitioner that is always trying to find the fastest, most effective way to release pain and restore function. "I've seen a fair number of gurus and master instructors in my day both in the more structured approaches as well as many of the more esoteric systems. I shy away from the word "amazing" when describing any good treatment technique, but after a series of actual patients were treated in this seminar and experienced positive results that were completely unexpected - by the patients as well as us! That's the only word to describe the results Dr. Kaufman's techniques yield - Simply amazing. It's interesting to hear the disclaimers about how Kaufman Techniques won't work on everybody. This is of course true in all healing methodologies. However, having practiced PNT and the other Kaufman Techniques for almost a year, I have yet to see a patient that did not get a positive response from treatment. I dare say that so far 100% of my patients have responded favorably and therapeutically in some measurable way. "In our field and in medicine, there are some methods that continue to be administered and are considered good with 40-50% efficacy; so to say that these methods are effective on 100% of my patients seems ridiculous, but it's true (at the time of this writing).
Moreover, I was already proficient and known as an elite practitioner that gets results where others do not. PNT has taken my game to a whole new level. I'm still waiting on my first non-

responder. As a natural skeptic, I still ask my patients, "are you sure?", when they report their results from only a few techniques in one session. But when range of motion improves, strength returns, functional levels increase; you have to acknowledge that a positive effect has occurred. There's your evidence.

Aside from that, the immediate results in subjective pain relief are nice too - and that's what most of our patients want in the first place. In essence, my patient outcomes are better and faster, and I have patients that are willing to pay out of pocket for this obvious higher level of care. Dr. Kaufman's work has helped me take my practice from a superb healing environment to an elite one. I would definitely be a patient in my clinic, so I'm satisfied...but I'm not done yet! This level of training is far from guru-based methods and placebo effects. There are real patients being treated and getting real results - objective and subjective! Interestingly, there was a patient with a cervical problem and another with a knee problem set for surgery; however, after this seminar, there are no surgeries planned. What an awesome experience, and I am excited to apply my new knowledge gained to further benefit my patients and all who want to be healthier, feel better, and move better!"

Wade Baskin, PT, DPT, RRT. Executive Director, GT Physical Therapy, Inc. Louisville, MS

" I'm getting clinical results that are better than ever before with a tiny fraction of the effort I was using before, (after attending the June 2012 class and adding the Sclerotome Techniques). The patients are happier than ever, and I have five new patients on the books for tomorrow. Who knew that following simple instructions could be so rewarding! The new Sclerotome work you introduced is really streamlining my ability to get people out of pain quickly. It's much more than an incremental change: Having this powerful new option has made working on low backs and shoulders so much easier. It's pure wizardry, based on solid science. Exceedingly gentle, yet it really gets the pain out fast! Muscle testing can impress people with before-and-after changes, but instantaneous pain relief is much harder to argue with. Thanks for the multi-faceted and multi-layered education! Also let me add my voice to the 47 others who are grateful to you and your cameraman for projecting the close-up videos of you at work. It really made it easier to learn.

The time you gave all of us shows how much you love this work, and your students. I will plan on being at next year's Bootcamp, for certain.

I first received the initial PNT DVDs from you about 5 years ago - then Manual Spinal Nerve Block. These immediately allowed us to access symptoms and conditions previously limited in response. I had studied 5 main chiropractic systems completely over my 25 years of practice (I mean completely, not just generic portions), which certainly helped, but your work began to take the help I could give, deeper and faster. It allowed me to greatly reduce the pain for my late wife (also a chiropractor) during her passing from pancreatic cancer, and since then has aided in my treatment of many hitherto inaccessible conditions. It has allowed me to treat myself of pain symptoms: low back, shoulder, wrist, headache. Posturally, I found application of this work far more effective than any of the chiropractic systems dedicated to postural adjustments (remarkable!). As I have integrated your work more and more during these years, I find myself mainly practicing according to your protocols, using, if at all, more the analysis of one or two of the chiropractic systems than the actual adjustments. I see many newborns and many elderly, and your work allows me to work with them all with increasing efficacy and in a completely pleasant way, i.e., not causing pain or discomfort. I now have all of your DVDs (I think). I really want to acknowledge the enormous contribution that you and your work have made in my life, and in the lives of all those with whom I come into contact. You will certainly receive an immense good karma for all of this. (Hope to make it sometime to a live seminar.) During this season of celebrating the miraculous, we'd certainly have to include the ones made possible through using the work in your Pain Control Patterns/ Visceral Impact Course. I worked on someone this morning who'd experienced a "minor" heart attack over the weekend. She felt a profound shift in her sense of well being after eliminating tenderness through some of the simplest techniques in the Pain Control Pattern course. Along with the mandibular reflex to help a chronic lateral atlas, she was a new woman! Having gotten used to major changes in shoulder ranges of motion using the paradoxical muscle techniques, it has been amazing to witness instantaneous doubling in shoulder flexion and abduction from even easier methods using single magical pain control points--without using needles.

*I appreciate the ability to positively and obviously influence peoples' breathing, digestive and other organ functioning. I have seen diabetics get back normal sensation in their feet in just a few visits. The brachial plexus sclerotome has helped many people with profound arm and hand numbness return to normal--often in one visit. Of course rapid musculoskeletal pain neutralization has become even more rapid and consistent with some of the more advanced techniques I've been learning. It is amazing to think that I only started using Pain Neutralization Technique a year and a half ago. I had a patient with intense, itching feet that would not allow her to sleep. This may have come from eating shellfish. Some sclerotome work and Pain Control Pattern work along with cranial work eliminated the symptoms within just a couple minutes." I'm also getting stellar results with knee, shoulder, neck, brachial plexus and other pains consistently. I have a very happy 94-year old patient. Her daughter originally brought her in to see me because knee pain on both sides was causing pain and mobility issues. Sometimes quality of life can be measured in terms of "How far can I walk?", and "Can I get in and out of a bathtub by myself?" After one visit using PNT, all her knee pain is gone. So, the patient then wanted to know whether I could help her hear better. We decided to go for it on the next visit. We increased her cervical rotation from 45 degrees to 90 on both sides, and got trigger points out of her cervical facets area, scalenes, SCMs and upper traps. The patient said that she could definitely hear more clearly. **She added that she can walk better and move her knee well enough to put on socks and pants.** I worked further on her neck today and her hearing continued to get clearer. The patient was even missing one hearing aid battery, and did OK. We worked on some post-shingles pain near the tailbone, and eliminated it using PCP and the Pain Grid."*
Stuart Marmorstein, DC Houston, TX

"I am The Worst at writing testimonials. This is because I'm too busy to write you a testimonial for every patient who is a success story, since that would be every patient I've treated since I started studying your work 6 or 7 years ago. I do not adjust or manipulate in any way - - I use only your techniques.

Of course there are the flashy "hero" patients: the spina bifida occulta patient, told she could never conceive a child, who carried a full-term, healthy baby after she received treatment with Kaufman Techniques; the patient born with all her abdominal organs on the outside of her body who endured multiple surgeries as a child and had constant pain all her life - - pain free after Abdominal PNT; several ptosed kidney patients helped with the psoas techniques; 5 different knee replacement patients, all with post-surgical RSD, all of whom had relief from pain with a variety of Kaufman Techniques; and many, many more.

But for me the truly amazing aspect of this work is how it helps my all-day every day patients. I practice in a ski resort town. I see a lot of knees, shoulders, concussions, whiplashes, low backs, groin pulls, and post-surgical discectomies, laminectomies, fusions, fractures, and the rest of the mayhem that goes with a population of extreme sports fanatics and World Cup teenagers.

I know you always say that these techniques don't work on everyone, but in 6 or 7 years of using your work I have never (that's never) had a patient whose pain I could not neutralize using one or more of your many terrific techniques.

So I know this doesn't follow your general testimonial format, but so far, in my personal experience, every patient I've ever treated with your techniques has had a personal miracle of pain and dysfunction relief that meant a lot to them and me – they are all testimonials to the efficacy of your work."
Valentina Lert, DC Telluride, CO

"I've used the left Stellate Ganglion Reflex (NOT the right) for pain in the abdomen from larger abdominal masses,, e.g. ovarian tumors, kidney and pelvic tumors, swollen legs."
David Walsh, MD Mobile, AL

"I've had many exciting responses, immediate elimination of pain and reduction of other symptoms. The techniques are quite effective in reducing inflammatory arthritis pain and swelling in my Lyme patients. In fact all my Lyme Patients this week reported improved mood and decreased pain. 31/32 success stories in 2 weeks. I've used the technique to reverse rapid onset of URI's and UTI's. Patients have found it very helpful in reducing pain, anxiety, de-

*pression, insomnia, and muscle spasms. Multiple chemical sensitivities and other allergies decreased. Chronic post abdominal surgery pain of many years disappeared in minutes. **This is what I went into medicine for! My prediction- PNT™ will change the course of medicine.***"
Karen Vrchota, MD Winona, MN

"I've had severe chronic thoracic spine pain for years. I get chiropractic manipulations, massage, intersegmental traction, even back rubs. Pain relief was always short lived from a few hours to a few days. Ever since my first seminar with you, 1 ½ years ago, the PNT used on my mid back has lasted all that time. Today there was only one spot that released in seconds and feels great now."
Bill Strempel, DC Denver, CO.

"In less than 5 minutes Dr. Kaufman rid me of trigger point pain in my trapezius that has been bothering me for over 20 years. I've had hundreds of massages, acupuncture – complete with electro stimulation, and chiropractic work, all of which would help somewhat but never got rid of the problem completely. Not only is my pain and tightness gone, but I witnessed many other class members gain almost instant relief as well. As a geographer, I appreciate Dr. Kaufman's command of the territory and landscape of the body. As a class participant, I appreciate the science behind the technique. As a body worker, I look forward to introducing my clients to this amazing work. As a skeptic, I am still in awe."
Rachel J. Brown, LMT Scotts Valley, CA

"I've had numerous patients on high doses of narcotics. Within a week or two of PNT treatment, they often don't need them any more. My wife has had rheumatoid arthritis and PNT is the only stuff that's kept her going. This is almost the only stuff she'd let me do to her. Just being able to treat your spouse so effectively is huge! I have associates with me virtually every time I come. I have yet to have anyone come (to a PNT seminar) that wasn't extremely happy they came. They go home and it changes their practice. This stuff works!"
Don Gay, DC Florence, CO.

Chapter 22

The future of PNT

From medical miracles that make patients and loved ones shed tears of joy, to poorly understood diseases that surprisingly show a significant positive response, PNT has so far walked many paths.

When judging the significance of advances in the health field, the impact a given innovation brings is likely measured by the following:

1) the potential reach each innovation has

2) how many lives can be bettered by it

3) how cost effective the innovation is

4) how profound of an improvement each innovation brings

5) how broad of a spectrum of disease processes such innovation impacts

6) how easy the implementation of said innovation is.

Over the last century medicine has seen many innovations with great impact. By far, PNT is the most "at hand" and one of the most significant innovation brought forward in the history of modern medicine. Wide in its potential reach like no other modern technology, a versed practitioner with a tooth brush and a change of underwear is all that is needed for PNT to reach every corner of the globe, requiring available only his or her hands and some space to carry out the treatment.

PNT has shown itself to be simple, effective and reproducible in an unprecedented wide variety of pathological conditions, either manifesting with pain or showing related signs (treatable areas of localized tenderness.) PNT has shown -to its practitioners and patients- what it has to offer in many areas where all other disciplines and approaches have little, if anything to add. Any health practitioner with basic knowledge of anatomy and pathophysiology can learn and implement the basic PNT techniques.

PNT's financial and biological cost-effectiveness will prove unsurpassed. With no known adverse effects, the practitioners' time and the time invested by the patient to get better are the only significant costs involved. A large number of reports have been presented through this book and exist beyond these pages. Many people with ailments for months or years, having spent countless resources looking for improvement, have found a life changing and problem solving experience in a few minutes or a short series of PNT treatments.

Furthermore, by its simplicity and reproducibility PNT is also leaping over many of the artificial disciplinary boundaries. The day will come when health practitioners will understand biochemistry and biophysics in the human body within the context of the flow of vital energy, within the context of the relationship to the environment, the self and the others, within the context of the cosmos, within the context of the individual and the overall consciousness.

PNT has the potential to be by far one of the most significant contributions to the healing arts in the history of medicine. While the list of milestones in modern medicine show a consistent increase and dependence on technological complexities, PNT brings forward the simplicity, beauty, elegance and reward of the simple healing hand. The contents of this book will spread. Readers will either seek to learn or to experience PNT. Their knowledge and experience will be shared with others. Each new experience will further the unfolding of PNT's full potential. PNT will become a primary tool in every health practitioner's hands.

Gaston Cornu- Labat, MD

www.tahomaclinicredmond.com

Epilogue to the first edition
By Stephen Kaufman, DC

This is likely the first time in history that a highly credentialed physician and surgeon has boldly gone where no physician and surgeon has gone before- he's written a book on the discoveries of a chiropractor. Many other board certified medical specialists have also contributed reports of their extraordinary successes using the Pain Neutralization Techniques™.

This is the forward at the end to my friend and colleague Dr Cornu-Labat's book on PNT, and indeed, "forward" is the direction we'd like to be moving.

As with any new ideas, discoveries, or viewpoints, we've met with resistance in trying to share the simple concept of eliminating chronic, intense myofascial pain quickly, for good, using easily learned neurological reflexes. The majority of practitioners in any field are resistant to any new idea that they didn't learn in school. This is to be expected, and certainly serves a purpose- many intriguing new concepts turn out not to be valid, over time.

However, as my friend Robert Rowen, MD editor of Second Opinion Newsletter, has said about Pain Neutralization Technique, "*the effect is so robust you don't need a double blind study to see that something amazing is happening here.*" Indeed, **every single time** I've presented PNT to an audience of medical or alternative practitioners, a large number of volunteers from the audience have been relieved of chronic, unrelenting pain of many types, which in every case has been unresponsive to previous medical, chiropractic, acupuncture, or other types of care. In some cases (not all), relief has been complete and long lasting, even after the one treatment that was performed on them.

It's important to note that results are often seen in **chronic pain-** by definition, pain becomes chronic because it has resisted all interventions to eliminate it. Acute pain may or may not go away tomorrow; chronic pain has steadily been here, and by definition will be here tomorrow.

PNT™ often works dramatically on acute pain as well, but since the natural history of an acute injury or condition is unknown it's harder to see the unique contribution of PNT to acute problems- they may have gone away on their own. Chronic problems do not disappear on their own, by definition.

There are 9 different, advancing levels of the PNT techniques, as of this writing, and no doubt many more will be discovered, over time. I've endeavored to make all these techniques widely available for licensed health care practitioners through seminars and DVD products, and information on these can be gotten from my website at **www.painneutralization.com** and our office, **303-756-9567 or 800-774-5078**.

When I began devising the techniques that became PNT, right up until today, my primary focus was on several things, the prime directives:

1. The techniques must be measurably, objectively effective, not theoretical- this means that they either immediately produce a reduction in an objective measure of pain, such as a trigger point or area on the body that's tender to pressure, or an observable increase in movement- e.g. if it hurts a patient to move his arm a certain way, that should improve immediately when a technique is applied.

2. The techniques must use minimal force; they must never be capable of causing harm.

3. They must produce clinical improvement, hopefully in a short number of sessions.

4. They must take a very short period of time to apply, almost always just a few seconds.

5. They must be so simple that each technique can be learned in less than a minute or two. (Although proper and deep understanding of the implications and theory behind each technique may of course take much longer.)

I think it speaks well that of the many dozens of procedures that have been developed over the past 20 years or so, each and every procedure remains effective and clinically useful. There are no techniques about which I would now say, "I changed my mind. It doesn't work." This of course can't be said about many drugs and other medical and even "holistic" procedures over the years, which are sometimes withdrawn from the market.

Early on there was an interest in the P.N.T techniques not only from the chiropractic profession, but from MDs, DOs, NDs, acupuncturists, PTs, DDSs, body workers, etc. Our live classes have become an amalgam with contributions from all these professions- that alone has been a source of warmth and joy for many attendees.

We've been fortunate in being able to expose over 5,000 doctors and other health care practitioners to at least some of the application of the many PNT techniques-tens of thousands of patients have been helped to some extent. This degree of interest and acceptance in such a short period of time far exceeded our hopes in the early stages of PNT.

As Gaston describes, the techniques have a much wider application than the relief of myofascial pain; there are many reports from doctors of successful PNT applications in a wide variety of visceral conditions including functional abdominal problems, irritable and inflammatory bowel conditions, GERD, hypertension, respiratory problems like asthma and bronchitis, allergies, fibromyalgia, some hormonal and gynecological conditions, esp. menstrual cramps, urinary conditions, vertigo, and emotional conditions such as P.T.S.D., unresolved emotional trauma, generalized anxiety disorders, etc. In all cases it's mandatory to rule out any type of pathology as a causative factor, and especially determine if medical care is needed.

In 1989, I set out intentionally to discover if there was a way to turn off pain using light fingertip pressure. After many years of being a doctor licensed to use chiropractic, acupuncture and many other modalities, I still could not consistently and lastingly target and turn off pain, or other symptoms. I knew a lot of techniques, but they were not specific for specific conditions. I had always suspected that "magic pain off switches" existed but had never seen or heard of them. Yet this was what patients really desperately needed, not the theory, philosophy and other junk that was constantly tossed at them. Patients needed and wanted their pain turned off, for good. Sure, most other procedures do this sometimes, but not consistently, as their therapeutic goal.

I had treated trigger points for many years with myofascial procedures and compression but I found this hard on the patient AND the doctor (it took a lot of force), and results were very often inconsistent and temporary. I thought there might be a way to gently TURN OFF trigger points, not just treat them, over and over again. If those trigger points were neutralized, many pain syndromes might likely improve or disappear.

The first intentional treatment I developed was the Vertigo Protocol. I had an 82 year old woman with constant, severe benign paroxysmal positional vertigo; she was so dizzy, she couldn't walk unaided. I applied a new soft tissue procedure to the upper part of her neck and her vertigo/dizziness stopped immediately.

This fortunate result lasted for 6 months- I needed to do one follow up treatment 6 months later as she developed some very slight vertigo again after that time. This technique has been used on 100s of patients with vertigo with a VERY high rate of success- some of these patients had had vertigo for more than 20 years.

The next intentional treatment I developed was for an employee with a very loudly clicking jaw every time she opened her mouth, of several years duration. After reviewing the anatomy of the TMJ I applied a very specific procedure, which immediately caused the jaw to stop clicking. This result was permanent on this patient. I've now treated many patients with clicking jaws, and many on film- we film all of our live seminars. In the majority of cases (not all) the clicking luckily stops immediately, even on camera.

It took until 2003 before I stumbled on the first reflex to instantly turn off myofascial trigger points and tender areas. Once I accidentally found the first one, in quick succession, I found half a dozen more reflexes, like a puzzle unraveling.

That was now 12 years ago. We've since been lucky to have discovered close to 100 different reflexes that can reliably reduce or eliminate the vast majority of myofascial trigger points. They also reduce tender areas in muscle, ligament or tendon that are sore to the touch (assuming there is no pathology present).

Of course not every patient or every condition responds, and many patients require a series of treatments to gain lasting benefit.

This morning I received a call from a practitioner who had read some of our material. She started the conversation by saying "I read that you can always turn off pain with one treatment." This was a grossly inaccurate misunderstanding on her part- I have never said that and never will!

There are patients who do not respond at all to these procedures, just like every other technique. There is no guarantee the PNT techniques will work in any particular case. Although many patients see rapid results in one or 2 visits, most patients require a few or a series of treatments for lasting benefit.

Having said that, we've accumulated many hundreds of reports from doctors and other practitioners of significant, often startling or unbelievable improvement, after one or more treatments. Even in the most difficult and stubborn of conditions. It would be foolish to deny that impressive results often occur rapidly in even the most stubborn of musculoskeletal conditions.

And as Dr. Cornu-Labat has said, when done correctly there is no possibility of injury from the gentle procedures involved. We are not attempting to move bones, force tissue to release, insert needles or other invasive procedures, but merely triggering neurological reflexes, with less force than is needed to routinely examine a patient or elicit a patellar tendon reflex, for example. We've now discovered scores of possible reflexes to immediately eliminate areas of palpatory pain (similar but not identical to so called "trigger points" as explained in chapter 3).

Stimulating the correct reflex will very frequently cause an immediate disappearance of painful, tender areas and increased range of motion related to the patient's individual symptoms, in the absence of any objective pathology. In many cases (again, not all), the patient's symptoms (headache, neck pain, back pain, sciatica, etc, etc) will also resolve.

Not every tender area responds to treatment; in some cases the effect doesn't last and the tender area keeps coming back. In some cases the tender area does disappear for good, but the patient's symptoms remain unchanged. These cases in my experience, and the reports of hundreds of PNT practitioners- are a small minority. Most patients show very significant objective and subjective improvement immediately, or in a short period of time. Of course when there is some type of pathology causing the patient's pain or disorder, the results will be less.

In school and for decades after graduation, most of what I saw were physical techniques that either often hurt the patient because they were too forceful, or were so light that they often had no discernable effect whatsoever. Patients themselves often became psychologically addicted to treatments they believed were helpful for them but seemed to me to do them no good over time. In my observation, almost all practitioners, medical and "alternative", seemed to operate under the following assumptions (which I strongly disagree with):

1. It's not possible to instantly eliminate objective signs of a patient's myofascial pain syndrome.

2. Any treatment of myofascial pain needs to be mechanical, not neural.

3. Since treatment is mechanical, a lot of force needs to be used to get results for the patient. This much force often ends up hurting the patient. Patients need to be hurt during treatment in order to get results.

4. Chronic pain can only be managed, not eliminated.

5. Lasting, even permanent pain relief within a short time is not even possible. The possibility of this was never even mentioned or considered in my chiropractic training.

All of these assumptions, so common in the treatment of myofascial pain, are considered false within the Pain Neutralization Technique™ paradigm. PNT treatment is gentle, and objective results (the disappearance of tender areas on the patient, improvement in range of motion of affected joints, muscles, and tendons) are generally immediate.

For the most part I've tried to let the 1000s of doctors practicing PNT speak for themselves and for me. This book contains a small percentage of their reports. I've tried to report only results that I or others have observed, and never claimed that PNT is good for everything, every condition or everyone. Many, many more reports can be found at our websites, www.painneutralization.com and www.pain2015.com.

I've never seen or heard of a significant side effect, though as with any-thing else, anytime you actually touch someone the possibility exists, no matter how remotely, for something to go wrong. I constantly counsel my students to use much less force than they're used to, and much less than they were trained to apply. I caution practitioners to be especially careful when applying even light, examination pressure to the abdomen or neck, front and back.

Nevertheless, occasionally students just cannot modify their early train-ing or overcome their (false) preconceptions of what's involved in a treatment- they use too much force. In spite of this, the techniques are so safe that to the best of my knowledge no lasting harm has ever been done.

The thousands of anecdotal reports from other doctors, and the more in depth reports from Dr Cornu-Labat, Dr Jawad Bhatti, MD, Dr. David Walsh, MD, Ran Kalif , L.Ac, Dr John Baird, MD, Reuben Mikel, DC, and many other doctors, don't constitute "proof" within the scientific community. It remains for researchers to conduct the necessary studies, which will undoubtedly come in time. The vast majority of other holistic procedures and even the majority of medical interventions also lack this strict, gold standard, double blind "proof", yet are in use by 1000s of practitioners every day. For now the reports of so many established and credentialed doctors will at least serve as extensive evidence that valid, important phenomena are taking place with the PNT techniques.

Although I read every doctor's report in this book years ago, I am literal-ly humbled and astounded as I reread them. I STILL find it almost unbe-lievable that so many patients, with so many diverse conditions, are helped so quickly, by so many doctors. And yet I see and hear about these results every single day. Last week I saw a woman regain full use of her arm and shoulder after 24 years of pain and extreme limitation of movement.

As overwhelming as the huge number of reports in this book may seem, I left out many hundreds of other cases, each one as dramatic as the ones in this book.

The secret reflexes that make up the Pain Neutralization Techniques™ have been hidden for thousands of years, waiting to be discovered. We're fortunate to find more and more of these reflexes, and get better and faster results, every year. It continues to humble and inspire awe in me, awe of the glory of creation and the glory of the Creator. As time goes on more and more doctors will take these basic procedures and add even more techniques to them.

Dr Cornu-Labat has done a great service to the many future patients that will read this book and be helped by PNT, and the many practitioners who will be thrilled to find such an easy, gentle way of greatly helping so many patients.

c. 2015 Stephen J. Kaufman, DC

www.painneutralization.com

303-756-9567

Appendix

PNT and the Parasympathetic Nervous System by Stephen Kaufman, DC

The control system for the human body is the autonomic nervous system. This is divided into the sympathetic and the parasympathetic nervous system. The Sympathetic Nervous System is responsible for fight or flight responses, muscular activity, the adrenal glands, and plowing forward. The Parasympathetic NS is responsible for sleep, rest, digestion, and healing.

The most recent developments in the Pain Neutralization Techniques, at the time this book is being written, are the PNT Brain Technique Reflexes™. These are procedures that are designed to rapidly reduce pain and many other symptoms, just like all the PNT techniques.

However, the Brain Technique Reflexes™ work by activating various portions of the brain to reduce reverberating neural loops that may be responsible for perpetuating chronic pain.

Pain may be maintained by local, spinal, or cortical tracts in the brain. The various types of PNT techniques work on different levels. The Brain Technique Reflexes™ employ concepts from psychology and neuroscience, along with ideas from Chinese medicine, to reduce or eliminate pain.

In addition, surprisingly, they often produce a PROFOUND state of immediate relaxation and anxiety reduction in a patient. We believe this indicates a powerful parasympathetic stimulation.

The following are a few of the many doctors' report we've received on the Brain Technique Reflexes™. The Brain Technique Reflexes™ have even been found to be effective for calming children with autism and attention deficit disorder.

"That's so weird" is all I've been hearing all day. I have been using the Brain Reflexes all day on patients and I can't believe how effective they are for stopping pain. Neck pain gone. Thumb pain gone. Hip pain gone. I even used a Brain Reflex™ while the patient did active right

cervical range of motion. It went from 60 degrees painful to 90 degrees pain free in 1 minute. I haven't had this much fun since I first used your PNT techniques 7 years ago.

"I come to the live seminars at least once a year to work with Dr. Kaufman. When I come, I am lucky enough to have Dr. Kaufman use his Respiratory Protocols to relieve chronic respiratory breathing difficulties since having complications with a total chest reconstruction when I was 13. Every time I get worked on I get significant lasting relief of shortness of breath. At the October 2014 class, Dr. Kaufman used the new Brain Reflexes™ to turn off several painful points along my diaphragm and psoas. My breathing immediately improved and to my surprise, my head was as clear as it has felt in years."
Reuben Mickel, DC Vancouver, WA

"I had a new female patient, 61, present with chronic, bilateral pain on top of the feet, with intermittent neuropathic pain in feet and toes. She was emotionally stressed out during intake. The PNT Brain Technique Reflex™ was administered for 2 minutes to support relaxation. Patient reported significant feeling of deep calmness and relaxation throughout her body within a minute. I then asked her to check how her feet felt. The pain was totally gone...in both feet! Wanting to confirm that the pain neutralization was holding, I had her walk around the room, and then down the hallway to see if the pain might come back. Her feet remained free of pain and she exclaimed: "You didn't even work on my feet and the pain is totally gone! How did you do that? Her feet have been free of pain for over a week as of this report. Since the October training, I have used the Brain Reflex Techniques™ on nearly every patient with "AMAZING" results! Every single person has reported a significant drop in stress level during treatment, and many have experienced site-specific, pain neutralization with only the Brain Technique Reflex stimulation. Combined with the other PNT techniques, the Brain Technique Reflex work has resulted in a huge improvement in progress for a couple of dozen patients already!"
Peter Goldberg, L.Ac. Greater Barrington, MA

"I had rotator cuff surgery on my left shoulder. I had torn the subscapularis muscle away from the proximal humerus and the surgeon reattached with 2 helix screws and cord. They also repaired the subscapu-

laris labrum and repaired the medial bicepital tendon. After PT, I was unable to reach behind my back or raise my arm in abduction past shoulder height. I had a severe trigger point in my left pectoral muscle that was eliminated using the new Brain Reflexes™. After one treatment by Dr. Kaufman, I was able to have full ROM in my left shoulder both in horizontal abduction and internal rotation."

Alan J. Weber, DC Moody, AL

"I volunteered as a patient for demonstration of the Brain Reflex for abdominal pain. I thought I had none. To my surprise, I had level 8 pain in the upper right quadrant. The Brain Reflex™ was used and the pain dissipated by 85%! I see a lot of shoulder issues and I get the "Wow!" factor constantly from doing PNT I've been in practice 40 years and I've done a lot of things, but PNT puts the "Amazing!" back into your practice! This was my 4ᵗʰ PNT seminar. Can't wait to put it to use on Monday. I love this stuff!"

Steve Evans, DC Longmont, CO

"I had bladder pain for about a week- it stopped when I had the Brain Technique Reflex™ done. I also had an amazing energy shift- it was almost mind boggling! Since the treatment I have a deeper sense of peace and calmness that just wasn't there before. I also had thumb pain for 8 months, feels 70% better after treatment. I've been a naturopath for 25 years, and I've been doing PNT for 10 years. My practice has gone from being nice, to being so much fun! Watching people's faces as they're amazed by PNT- there's not one day that goes by that I don't laugh a good part of the day (with my patients, at the results from PNT)."

Peggy Wells N.D. Matthews, NC

"I've had abdominal pain and discomfort for 3 years. I've had significant improvement the last year with PNT. This morning, Dr. Kaufman treated me with the new Brain Technique Reflexes™ and it's now totally gone. I had an energy shift through my whole body- it's awesome stuff!"

Steve R. Vought Silbis, IL

"At the October 2014 seminar, Dr. Kaufman worked on me using his new Brain Technique Reflexes™. I've had neck pain for about 2 years during which I have tried multiple soft tissues modalities and chiropractic work with no lasting effect. When I sat up after the treatment, Dr.

Kaufman was saying something about feeling different, but I was in such a mental fog and my body was being washed by endorphins that it was difficult to make a response. After allowing about 15 minutes for my nervous system to settle down, I realized how relaxed my entire body was and amazingly PAIN FREE!!! I woke up the next morning, and my hip didn't hurt! I slept all night. Also, the pain in my thumb is still gone the next day. PNT has made a PHENOMENAL impact on my practice. I use it on every single client."
Debra Vought, L.M.T. Silbis, IL

The PNT Family of Techniques

Throughout this book many doctors have mentioned various types of PNT techniques. Pain Neutralization Technique includes various levels developed since 2000, as follows;

Pain Neutralization Techniques™-Level 1. This is the foundation class that every practitioner starts with. These are the first reflexes that eliminate trigger points on the spot with light touch. Many of these reflexes are hypothesized to work by triggering Golgi tendon reflexes in various ways, on the tendons and muscle bellies, in both agonist and antagonist muscles.

Level 1 also introduces PNT Meridian and Tissue Bending™.

The Manual Spinal Nerve Block Techniques™-Level 2- manual spinal nerve blocks are mediated through several types of spinal cord reflexes. With these techniques the patient's pain can be treated from various areas of the spine, wherever on the body the pain occurs. Visceral and abdominal pain can often be helped with these techniques. Many cases of post surgical pain, and very long standing abdominal, intestinal and pelvic pain have cleared up with these techniques. Radicular pain such as sciatica, causalgia, and arm/shoulder syndromes also respond well.

The Manual Spinal Nerve Blocks take the THEORY elaborated in chiropractic and acupuncture meridian theory and make them REALITY.

The Pain Elimination Grid™ Family of Techniques- Level 3- these techniques are the simplest, most rapidly effective techniques imaginable for turning off pain. The most widely accepted theory of chronic pain is the Melzack Wall Gate Theory of Pain. The Grid Family of Techniques, based on that theory, has opened a new universe of possibilities in simple, drug free, hands only pain control. There have been literally thousands of reports of instant relief from chronic pain

The Pain Elimination Grid also easily addresses pain and dysfunction in ligaments, menisci, bursa, bones and boney surfaces, and joints as well as muscles, tendons, nerve pain, and visceral and soft tissue problems. The techniques may eliminate chronic pain from scar tissue. They are applicable almost anywhere in the body.

The Pain Control Patterns™ -Level 4- are the most advanced Meridian Bending techniques, including the master quadrant controls. They also include new procedures for greatly enhancing lymphatic activity, the Visceral Impact procedures.

The Sclerotome Deep Pain Procedures™ -Level 5- Sclerotomes are maps of a patient's pain areas, arising from deep structures related to spinal nerves. The Sclerotome Techniques turn off a patient's pain right away, often for good, by interrupting the feedback from reverberating neural circuits in the sclerotomes.

PNT Level 6- procedures address the Adrenal and Sympathetic Nervous Systems.

PNT Level 7- the PNT Brain Technique Reflexes™. These reflexes stimulate areas of the brain that are involved in the perpetuation of persistent chronic pain, making use of dual attention stimuli procedures that are recognized in the field of psychology and neuroscience.

PNT Level 8- Brain Technique Reflexes Volume 2

PNT Level 9- Brain Technique Reflexes Volume 3